ATLAS OF STRABISMUS

ATLAS OF STRABISMUS

Gunter K. von Noorden, M.D.

Professor of Ophthalmology, Baylor College of Medicine, and Director of
Ophthalmology, Texas Children's and St. Luke's Episcopal Hospitals,
Houston, Texas

A. Edward Maumenee, M.D.

Professor of Ophthalmology and Director, The Wilmer Institute of Ophthalmology,
The Johns Hopkins University, School of Medicine, and Hospital,
Baltimore, Maryland

SECOND EDITION
325 illustrations in 124 figures, 34 in color, by Robert B. Wingate, D.Sc., F.R.S.A.

The C. V. Mosby Company

Saint Louis   1973

Second edition

Copyright © 1973 by The C. V. Mosby Company

*All rights reserved. No part of this book may be reproduced
in any manner without written permission of the publisher.*

Previous edition copyrighted 1967

Printed in the United States of America

International Standard Book Number 0-8016-5251-0

Library of Congress Catalog Card Number 72-87643

Distributed in Great Britain by Henry Kimpton, London

Affectionately dedicated to

Betty and Anne

Foreword

In a delightful little book, *Friends and Fiddlers,* Catherine Drinker Bowen describes the urge that induced her to write about playing chamber music as follows: " . . . a life lived intimately with music has made me only the more desirous to shape this intimacy into words; like a lover, I burn to declare myself."

It is easy to understand why these authors have committed themselves to the task of producing this book on strabismus. Their intimacy with the oculomotor mechanism is such that they too must have "burned to declare" themselves. They had to write this book. And that is both well for them and extremely fortunate for us.

Dr. von Noorden has spent his ophthalmologic life, including a residency with Hermann Burian, thinking and experimenting in the various phases of comitant strabismus, particularly its sensory aspects. In a few short years his writings have brought him the respect and admiration of his confreres in this field. Dr. Maumenee brings to the combined effort the vast experience of the Director of the Wilmer Institute and the deserved reputation of one of the best minds in ophthalmology in the world.

The authors have modestly described and titled this as an atlas, and to the extent that it is profusely illustrated the title is correct. But it is hardly adequate, and were I involved with the sale of the book I would hasten to let prospective readers know that it contains a text quite commensurate with, if not of greater value than, the illustrations. An atlas is generally conceived as a collection of pictures with captions; a textbook, a verbal account with illustrations. This book lies somewhere between the two. It could have been a textbook written by that famous Chinese sage who said, "One illustration is worth a thousand words." At any rate, it is an extremely satisfying and efficient means of learning the methods one should employ to examine patients with oculomotor difficulties. To explain to someone how to do a thing is best accomplished by the use of pictures, and that is why this book is so effective—the pictures show you how to do it.

The pedagogic know-how of the authors is evident in the logical way the material has been presented. Essentially a book of instruction, it commences with a broad base of anatomy and physiology, emphasizing those features that have clinical significance. Even in this first section the practical applications are stressed. For example, the definition of Hering's law is followed by a description of secondary deviation in cases of muscle paralysis and inhibitional palsy of the contralateral antagonist of the paralyzed muscle. Tests differentiating heterophoria from heterotropia are graphically described. An evaluation of the sensory status of the patient is next considered, again with emphasis on how to perform the tests. Some of these tests have only recently been described, such as the Bagolini striated glass test and the Cüppers test for retinal correspondence. Even the more experienced ophthalmologist will find condensed and simplified accounts of subjects for which he hopefully believed he might find sufficient time someday to read in the original. Occasionally the authors suggest new lines of thinking, as when they point out the fact that the afterimage test for the presence of ARC is only valid, strictly speaking, if one has previously checked the fixation pattern with the Visuscope. This is the first suggestion I have seen that our usual methods of determining the fixation of an eye are inadequate for the purposes of discovering anomalous retinal correspondence. When one comes to think about it, the older methods are quite crude, especially when one remembers that a shift of fixation of an eye of less than 2 degrees cannot be detected by visual observation, and yet a shift of 2 degrees off the fovea reduces the visual acuity from 20/15 to around 20/50.

Following the discussion of the sensory components of strabismus is an evaluation of the motor status, and finally the description and illustration of some forms of strabismus. Treatment, while not stressed, is included in many sections; for example, the authors' preference in the surgical management of the A and V patterns.

This book epitomizes the facts of strabismus without too much waving of the rallying flags of theory, which are admittedly alluring but very confusing to the young ophthalmologist whose chief interest is to know how to find out what the patient's trouble is.

Francis Heed Adler, M.D.

Preface to second edition

In preparing the second edition of this book, the concept of improving and clarifying the text and some of the illustrations was our main consideration. New illustrations were added to enhance the teaching value, and additional key references were included. We are grateful to the domestic and foreign reviewers of the first edition for their suggestions and constructive criticisms. Our thanks also go to readers who took the time and trouble to write their suggestions and, in some instances, direct our attention to the fortunately few errors that inadvertently crept into the first edition. These have been corrected.

We hope that the second edition will enjoy the same acceptance as the first in serving its primary purpose—to provide the beginner with a useful introduction into one of the most complex fields of ophthalmology.

Gunter K. von Noorden
A. Edward Maumenee

Preface to first edition

The diagnosis of strabismus, including its sensory adaptations and motor characteristics, depends on thorough examination and correct interpretation of a great number of subjective and objective tests. In recent years our diagnostic resources have become enlarged and refined by new procedures, and new information on the nature of sensory adaptations in strabismus has necessitated a different interpretation of some of the older tests. Information on this subject is scattered throughout national and world literature and cannot easily be assembled by the ophthalmologist.

This atlas does not attempt to fill the need for a comprehensive textbook on strabismus; rather it illustrates and provides basic information for the examination and diagnosis of strabismic patients in the light of present knowledge. It is not written for the expert but is designed primarily for the ophthalmologist-in-training, for the practicing ophthalmologist who is confronted by diagnosis of complex muscle problems only occasionally, and for the orthoptist.

Many diagnostic procedures to which the expert is accustomed are not included in this book. We have not endeavored to be comprehensive, but rather to include and describe only those tests that in our experience have proved most practical, do not require elaborate equipment and extensive space, and are frequently employed in our Motility Clinic.

It would exceed the purpose of this atlas to provide a complete list of references pertaining to all subjects under discussion. However, a few references have been selected for the student of strabismus who desires additional information on the more recently introduced tests.

We hope this atlas may be of assistance to our colleagues in recognizing and analyzing strabismus problems, and that it will aid the understanding of the basis and interpretation of the described diagnostic procedures.

We are deeply indebted to Robert B. Wingate, without whose imaginative and artistic drawings this atlas could not have been completed. We also wish to express our gratitude to the Wilmer Photography Service for their cooperation, to David Andrews for his editorial suggestions and for preparing the index, and to Patricia Bond for typing the manuscript.

Gunter K. von Noorden
A. Edward Maumenee

Contents

I. Anatomy and physiology of extraocular muscles

ACTION OF EXTRAOCULAR MUSCLES

Under normal conditions no extraocular muscle ever contracts alone. Innervational and inhibitional impulses flow simultaneously to all muscles. The action of a muscle depends on the angle between its *plane* (determined by the center of rotation of the globe and the centers of origin and insertion of the muscle) and the *optical axis* of the eye. It follows that the action of the muscle may vary according to the position of the globe in the orbit.

ACTION OF EXTRAOCULAR MUSCLES—cont'd
Horizontal rectus muscles

In the horizontal rectus muscles the muscle plane coincides with the optical axis when the eye is in primary position. The action of the medial rectus is one of pure adduction and the action of the lateral rectus is one of pure abduction when the eye is in primary position. Secondary actions of the horizontal rectus muscles when the eye is in other than primary position are clinically of less importance.

Figure 1
A Action of the medial rectus muscle (adduction).
B Action of the lateral rectus muscle (abduction).

Vertical rectus muscles

Figure 2. Superior rectus.
A When the eye is in primary position, the muscle plane of the superior rectus forms an angle of 23° with the optical axis. In this position the superior rectus elevates the globe. Secondary actions include incycloduction and adduction.
B As the eye moves into adduction, the superior rectus becomes less of an elevator and more of an adductor and incycloductor. In 67° adduction the superior rectus would become the exclusive source of incycloduction while still having adductive power. The position of 67° is chosen for theoretical reasons only; the eye is never adducted that far.
C In 23° abduction the superior rectus becomes a pure elevator. In this position the muscle plane coincides with the optical axis.

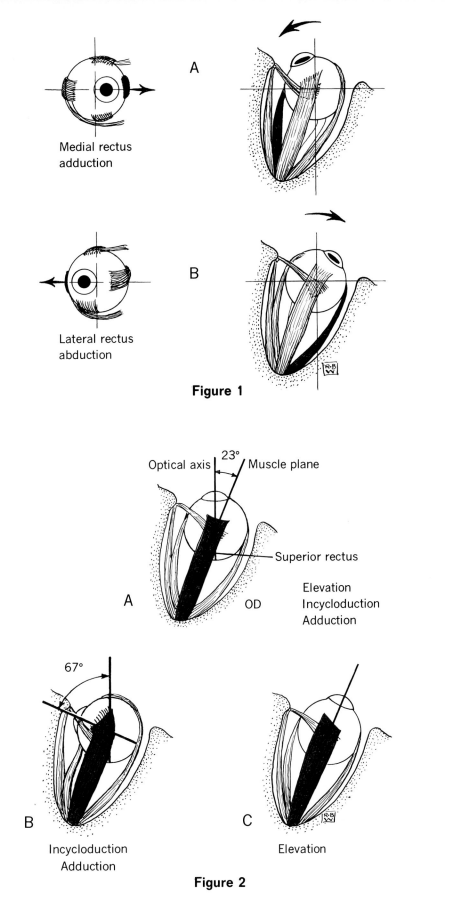

Medial rectus
adduction

Lateral rectus
abduction

Figure 1

Optical axis   23°   Muscle plane

Superior rectus

A   Elevation
                        OD   Incycloduction
                                     Adduction

67°

Incycloduction
Adduction   Elevation

B   C

Figure 2

3

Vertical rectus muscles—cont'd

Figure 3. Inferior rectus.

A With the eye in primary position the inferior rectus forms an angle of 23° with the optical axis. Thus the relationship between muscle plane and optical axis is identical to that of the superior rectus. In primary position the inferior rectus depresses the globe; secondary actions include excycloduction and adduction.

B As the eye moves into adduction, the inferior rectus becomes less of a depressor and more of an excycloductor and adductor. In 67° adduction it would become the exclusive source of excycloduction and aid adduction. However, the eye is never adducted that far.

C In 23° abduction the inferior rectus becomes a pure depressor; in this position the muscle plane coincides with the optical axis.

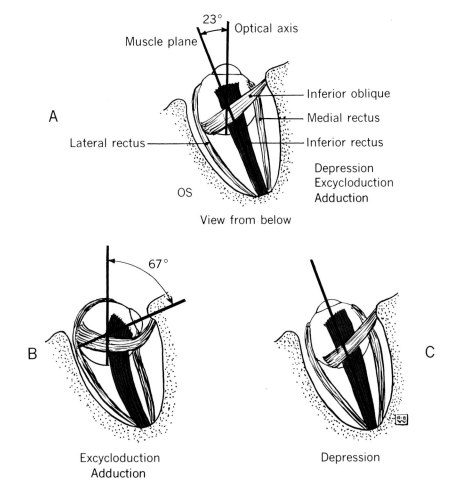

23°

Optical axis

Muscle plane

A

Inferior oblique

Medial rectus

Inferior rectus

Lateral rectus

Depression
Excycloduction
Adduction

OS

View from below

67°

B

Excycloduction
Adduction

C

Depression

Figure 3

ACTION OF EXTRAOCULAR MUSCLES—cont'd

Oblique muscles

Figure 4. Superior oblique.

A When the eye is in primary position, the muscle plane of the superior oblique muscle forms an angle of 54° with the optical axis. In this position the principal action of the superior oblique is one of incycloduction; secondary actions include abduction and depression.

B When the globe is adducted 54°, the optical axis coincides with the muscle plane. In this position the muscle still acts as an incycloductor, but its vertical action becomes more significant.

C When the globe is abducted, the superior oblique is primarily an incycloductor and secondarily an abductor.

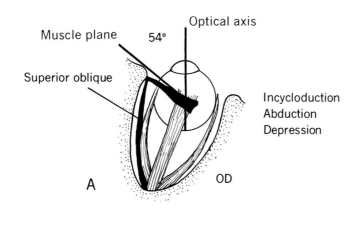

Muscle plane 54° Optical axis

Superior oblique

Incycloduction
Abduction
Depression

A   OD

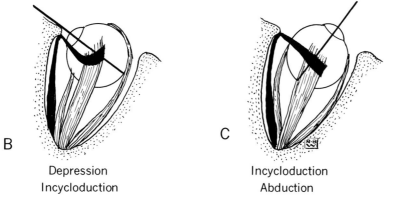

B

Depression
Incycloduction

C

Incycloduction
Abduction

Figure 4

7

Oblique muscles—cont'd

Figure 5. Inferior oblique.

A When the eye is in primary position, the muscle plane of the inferior oblique forms an angle of 51° with the optical axis. In this position the principal action of the inferior oblique is one of excycloduction; secondary actions include abduction and elevation.

B When the eye is adducted 51°, the optical axis approaches the muscle plane. The muscle still acts as an excycloductor but its action as an elevator becomes more significant.

C In abduction the inferior oblique acts primarily as an excycloductor and secondarily as an abductor.

The foregoing descriptions summarize the classic analysis of extraocular muscle actions. However, modern views have challenged this concept. Mathematical-geometric analysis of the muscle action[1] and experimental work with monkeys[2] have shown that the vertical rectus muscles remain the main elevators and depressors and that the primary action of the oblique muscles is one of cycloduction regardless of whether the globe is abducted or adducted. Although clinical evidence contradicts this newer hypothesis, many of the arguments presented by its proponents are convincing. Thus it may be necessary to change our present concepts if more data supporting this view become available.

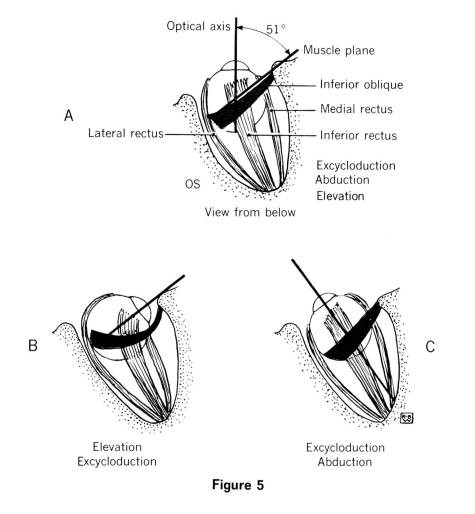

A

Optical axis   51°

Muscle plane

Inferior oblique

Medial rectus

Lateral rectus

Inferior rectus

Excycloduction
Abduction
Elevation

OS

View from below

B

Elevation
Excycloduction

C

Excycloduction
Abduction

Figure 5

9

TOPOGRAPHY OF EXTRAOCULAR MUSCLES

Figure 6

Illustration of the topographic relationships of the extraocular muscles to each other and to adjacent structures.

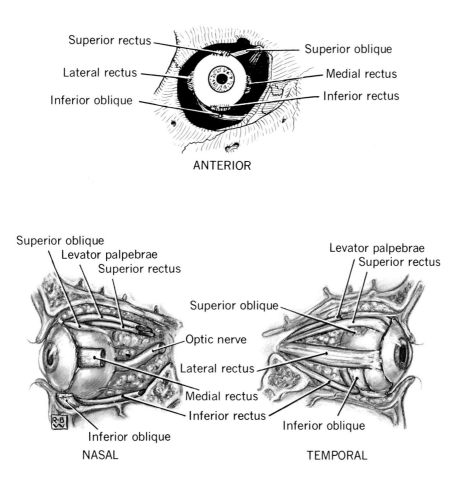

Superior rectus
Lateral rectus
Inferior oblique
Superior oblique
Medial rectus
Inferior rectus

ANTERIOR

Superior oblique
Levator palpebrae
Superior rectus

Optic nerve
Lateral rectus
Medial rectus
Inferior rectus
Inferior oblique

NASAL

Levator palpebrae
Superior rectus
Superior oblique

TEMPORAL

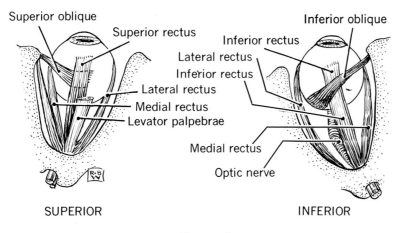

Superior oblique
Superior rectus
Lateral rectus
Medial rectus
Levator palpebrae

SUPERIOR

Inferior oblique
Inferior rectus
Lateral rectus
Inferior rectus
Medial rectus
Optic nerve

INFERIOR

Figure 6

11

SPIRAL OF TILLAUX

Figure 7
Demonstrating the width of the tendinous insertion and the distance of the insertion in millimeters from the limbus of the four rectus muscles of the right eye. The medial rectus tendon is closest to the limbus; the superior rectus is farthest. By connecting circularly the insertions of the tendons, one obtains the spiral of Tillaux. Note that the insertions of the superior and inferior rectus muscles are not entirely parallel to the limbus and that the distance between their lateral aspects and the limbus is greater than the distance between their medial aspects and the limbus.

PRIMARY AXES OF THE GLOBE

Figure 8
Movements of the globe occur around three primary axes. Each axis passes through the center of rotation and forms a right angle with the others.

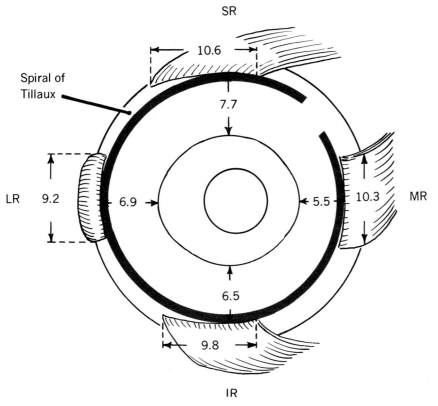

Figure 7

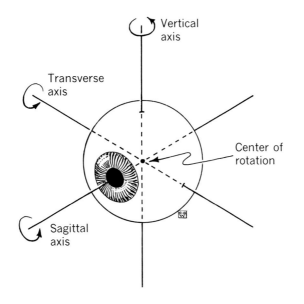

Figure 8

13

MONOCULAR AND BINOCULAR EYE MOVEMENTS
Movements of a single eye—ductions

Figure 9
A Horizontal movements of a single eye around the vertical axis.
B Vertical movements of a single eye around the transverse axis.
C Cyclorotational ("wheel-rotational") movements of a single eye around the sagittal (anteroposterior) axis.

14

Right eye

A

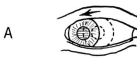 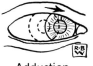

Abduction   Adduction

B

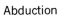 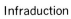

Supraduction   Infraduction

C

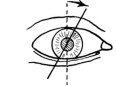 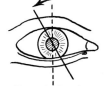

Incycloduction   Excycloduction

Figure 9

15

MONOCULAR AND BINOCULAR EYE MOVEMENTS—cont'd

Movements of both eyes—versions and vergences

Synchronous and symmetric movements of both eyes in same direction —versions (conjugate movements):

Figure 10
A Movements of both eyes to the right and to the left.
B Movements of both eyes up and down.
C Wheel-rotational movements of both eyes around an anteroposterior axis to the right and to the left.

Synchronous and symmetric movements of both eyes in opposite directions —vergences (disjugate movements):

Figure 11
A Convergence and divergence.
B OD moves up while OS moves down and vice versa. Positive vertical divergence is synonymous with right sursumvergence; negative vertical divergence is synonymous with right deorsumvergence.
C Both eyes rotate nasally or temporally around an anteroposterior axis. Incyclovergence is synonymous with conclination; excyclovergence is synonymous with disclination.

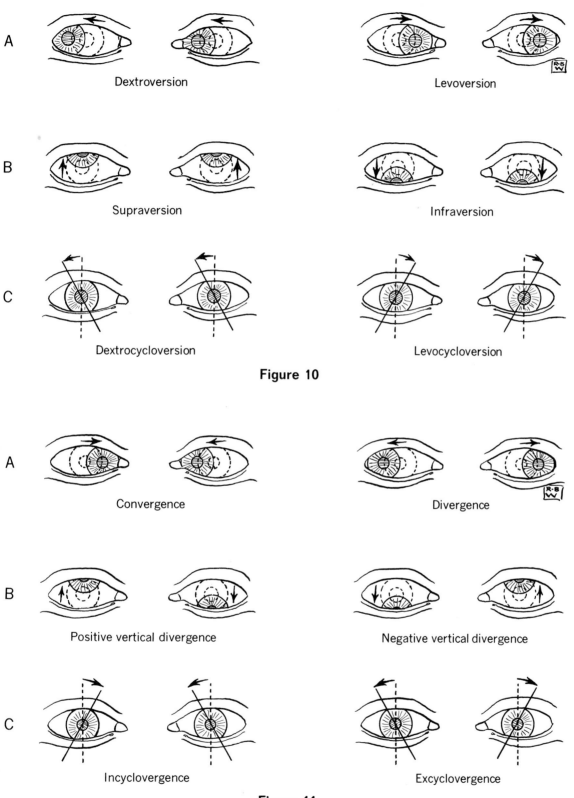

A   Dextroversion   Levoversion

B   Supraversion   Infraversion

C   Dextrocycloversion   Levocycloversion

Figure 10

A   Convergence   Divergence

B   Positive vertical divergence   Negative vertical divergence

C   Incyclovergence   Excyclovergence

Figure 11

17

DIAGNOSTIC POSITIONS OF GAZE

Examination of the ocular positions in the main fields of action of each of the twelve extraocular muscles is an essential step in the work-up of the strabismic patient. (For further details, see the following discussions.)

Examination of ductions can indicate weakness or overaction of one or several muscles. Examination of versions determines whether a strabismus is comitant (the angle of deviation does not change significantly in the various diagnostic positions) or incomitant (the angle varies according to the direction of gaze).

In order to detect deficiencies of ocular motility in extreme positions of gaze it is important to remove the patient's spectacles when examining ductions and versions.

The prism-cover test, carried out with either eye fixating in the diagnostic positions, often makes it possible to detect the paretic muscle in complicated problems of vertical or oblique muscles, the deviation being greatest in the field of action of the paretic muscle and with the paretic eye fixating. Measurements of the deviation with the eyes in the straight-up and straight-down position can reveal A or V patterns in horizontal strabismus.

Figure 12
The nine diagnostic positions of gaze.

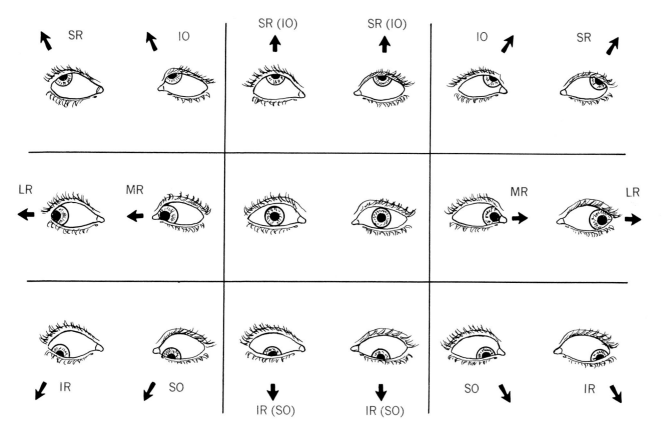

Figure 12

19

HERING'S LAW OF EQUAL INNERVATION

According to Hering, equal and simultaneous innervation flows to synergistic muscles (or muscle groups) concerned with the desired direction of gaze. This law applies to all voluntary and to some involuntary eye movements, and its validity has been confirmed electromyographically.

Hering's law in versions, vergences, and cycloversions

Figure 13

A During levoversion the right medial and the left lateral rectus muscles receive an equal and simultaneous flow of innervation.

B During convergence the right and left medial rectus muscles receive equal and simultaneous innervation.

C When the head is tilted to the left, the muscle groups concerned with excycloduction of OD and with incycloduction of OS receive equal and simultaneous innervation. However, inclination of the head is only partially compensated for by wheel-rotations of the eyes.

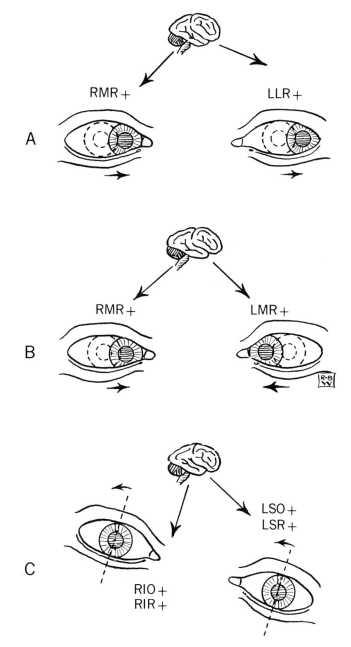

Figure 13

HERING'S LAW OF EQUAL INNERVATION—cont'd

Clinical applications of Hering's law

Primary and secondary deviation:

The greatest practical significance of Hering's law is its application to the diagnosis of paralytic strabismus. Since the amount of innervation flowing to both eyes is always determined by the fixating eye, the angle of deviation will vary, depending on whether the patient fixates with the sound eye (primary deviation) or paretic eye (secondary deviation). Thus measurements of the deviation in the diagnostic positions, with each eye fixating in turn, are of paramount importance in detecting the paretic muscle or muscle group when the strabismus is incomitant.

Figure 14

A In a case of right abducens paresis, normal innervation is required to move the left (normal) eye in adduction during dextroversion. OD does not follow beyond the midline, since the normal amount of innervation (+) required by OS is not sufficient to overcome the paresis of the RLR. The resulting horizontal deviation is called primary deviation.

B When the paretic right eye fixates, excessive amounts of innervation (+ + +) are required to execute abduction during dextroversion. According to Hering's law, the same impulses will be transmitted to the normal LMR, resulting in excessive adduction OS. *This secondary deviation is greater than the primary deviation.* (The thickness of the arrows symbolizes excessive innervation.)

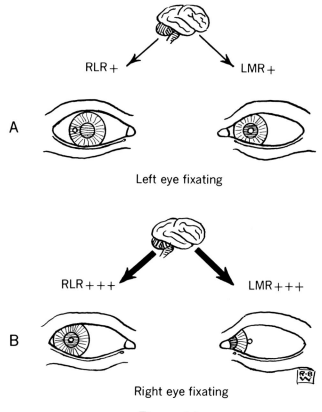

A

Left eye fixating

B

Right eye fixating

Figure 14

23

HERING'S LAW OF EQUAL INNERVATION—cont'd

Clinical applications of Hering's law—cont'd

Inhibitional palsy of contralateral antagonist:

The antagonist of a paretic muscle will require less than normal innervation to move the eye in its field of action, since the normal tonus of its paretic opponent will be decreased. Thus, according to Hering's law, the yoke muscle of the antagonist of the paretic muscle will receive less than normal innervation and may be apparently underacting when the paretic eye is fixating. This phenomenon has led to confusion between paresis of the superior oblique of one eye and the superior rectus in the fellow eye. It occurs *only* when the paretic eye is fixating and disappears after occlusion of the paretic eye.

Figure 15. Paresis of right superior oblique muscle.

A **Paretic eye fixating.** There will be little or no vertical difference between the two eyes in the right (uninvolved) field of gaze (**1**) and (**4**).

In primary position (**3**) a left hypotropia may be present, since the right elevators require less innervation and thus the left elevators will receive less than normal innervation.

When looking to the left and up (**2**), the RIO needs less than normal innervation (+) to elevate OD, since its opponent, the RSO, is paretic. Consequently, its yoke, the LSR, will be apparently underacting (+), and pseudoptosis with pseudoparesis of the LSR will be present.

When looking toward the field of action of the paretic muscle (**5**), maximal innervation is required to move OD down during adduction (+ + +), and thus the LIR (contralateral synergist) will be overacting.

B **Sound eye fixating.** There will be no vertical difference in the right field of gaze (**1** and **4**).

In primary position (**3**) OD is elevated because of unbalanced elevators.

When looking up and left (**2**), the RIO shows marked overaction, since its antagonist is paretic and there is contracture of the unopposed muscle. Note that pseudoparesis of LSR is no longer present. (Compare with Figure 15, **A, 2.**)

When looking down and left (**5**), normal innervation required by the fixating normal eye does not suffice to fully move the paretic eye.

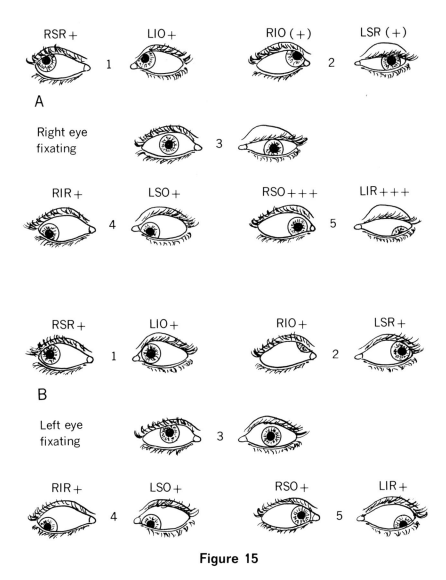

Figure 15

SHERRINGTON'S LAW OF RECIPROCAL INNERVATION

According to Sherrington's law, muscle contraction does not increase simultaneously in opposed muscles, nor does it decrease simultaneously in opposed muscles. In ocular motility this implies that under normal conditions an increased contraction of an extraocular muscle is accompanied by diminution of contractile activity in its antagonist. Under pathologic conditions exceptions to Sherrington's law may occur; they consist of rhythmic co-contractions of medial and lateral rectus muscles of the same eye (retractory nystagmus) or co-contraction of medial and lateral rectus muscles of the same eye on attempted adduction (Duane's retraction syndrome).

Figure 16

A On levoversion, increased contraction (+) of the RMR and LLR is accompanied by decreased tonus (**o**) of the antagonistic RLR and LMR.

B Increased activity of both medial rectus muscles and decreased tonus of both lateral rectus muscles during convergence.

C Contraction and relaxation of opposing muscle groups on dextrocycloversion when the head is tilted to the left shoulder.

26

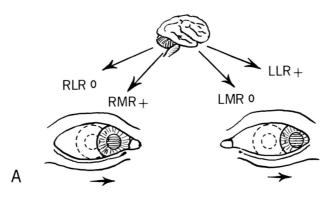

A

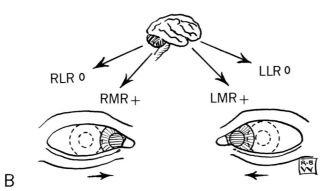

B

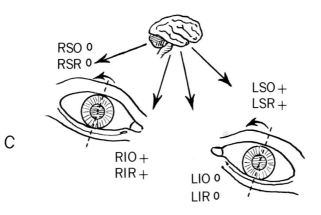

C

Figure 16

27

II. Pseudostrabismus

PSEUDOESOTROPIA

Prominent epicanthal fold

A prominent epicanthus may obscure some or all of the usually visible nasal aspects of the globe, thus giving the false impression that esotropia is present (Figure 17). In most infants the originally flat nasal bridge develops as they grow older, lifting the excessive epicanthal skin and correcting the condition.

The negative angle kappa is discussed on page 32.

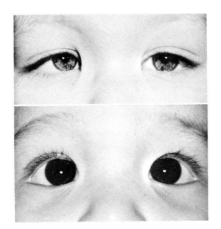

Figure 17

PSEUDOEXOTROPIA

Hypertelorism

Wide separation of the two eyes may occur as a result of disproportional growth of the facial bones or as a primary deformity. Such persons may appear exotropic, even though in fact the eyes are straight—although exotropia does occur in congenital dysostoses accompanied by hypertelorism.

Figure 18
A healthy 9-year-old girl with an interpupillary distance of 68 mm. Positive angle kappa OD. Pseudoexotropia.

Figure 19
A patient with acrocephalosyndactylia (Apert's disease). Although this deformity is frequently associated with exotropia, this boy had orthophoria at both near and distance. Pseudoexotropia.

The positive angle kappa and ectopic macula are discussed on pages 32 and 34, respectively.

PSEUDOHYPERTROPIA

Facial asymmetries or orbital tumors that displace the globe vertically may simulate vertical ocular deviations.

Figure 20
This 17-year-old boy had marked facial asymmetry. The left palpebral fissure was higher than the right, and an LHT* appeared to be present. The cover test actually revealed an RHT of 7$^\triangle$.

---

*The commonly used abbreviations LHT for left hypertropia, RHT for right hypertropia, ET for estropia, and XT for exotropia will be employed throughout this book.

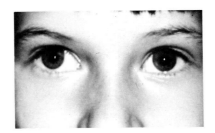

Figure 18

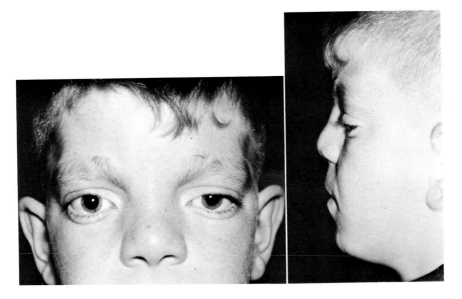

Figure 19

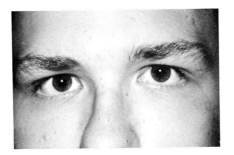

Figure 20

31

DIFFERENTIAL DIAGNOSIS OF DECENTERED CORNEAL LIGHT REFLEX

The Hirschberg and prism reflex tests and the determination of the angle of strabismus on the amblyscope depend on the position of the corneal light reflex. In addition to a heterotropia a number of other conditions may lead to decentration of the corneal light reflex and must be considered in order to correctly interpret tests based on the light reflex.

Angle kappa

The angle kappa is defined as the angle between the *visual line* (line connecting the point of fixation with the nodal points and the fovea) and the *pupillary axis* (line through the center of the pupil perpendicular to the cornea). This angle is actually formed at the anterior nodal point. In clinical practice the angle is measured at the center of the pupil (Figure 21, *A*). It is called positive when the light reflex is displaced nasally and negative when it is displaced temporally (Figure 21, *B*). A positive angle kappa of up to 5° is physiologic in emmetropic eyes.

Objective measurement: A muscle light is moved on a perimeter arc until the light is centered on the cornea, while the patient fixates on the center mark on the perimeter. The difference in the position of the muscle light and center mark is indicated in degrees of arc and constitutes the angle kappa.

Subjective measurement: The patient looks at the center spot (such as the zero mark or dog in Figure 21, *C*) of slides with angular calibrations, which are inserted into the major amblyoscope. If the examiner notes that the light reflex is decentered, the patient is requested to look from number to number until the light is centered. The number seen by the patient indicates the angle kappa in degrees of arc.

Significance of angle kappa: A positive angle kappa may simulate an exodeviation (Figure 18), and a negative angle kappa may simulate an esodeviation. Conversely, strabismus may be less apparent and escape detection by the parents when a large positive angle kappa is associated with esotropia, or a large negative angle with exotropia.

Tests for the detection of manifest strabismus that may be obscured by a large angle kappa will be discussed subsequently.

A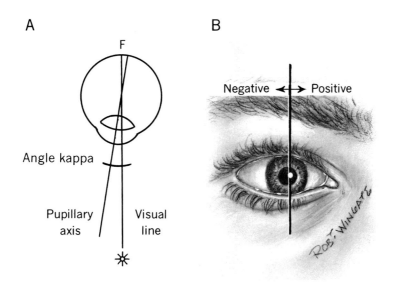

B

C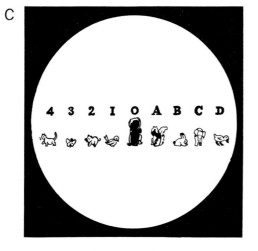

Figure 21

DIFFERENTIAL DIAGNOSIS OF DECENTERED CORNEAL LIGHT REFLEX—cont'd

Eccentric fixation

When the deviated eye is amblyopic and the light reflex remains decentered upon covering of the sound eye, eccentric fixation is usually present.

Figure 22
A Temporally decentered light reflex OS; VOS: 5/200.
B Light reflex OS remains decentered when OD is occluded.
C Series of fixation photographs of OS reveal fixation with a retinal area 1 disc diameter nasal to the optic disc. Each black circle represents a position of the fixation target on the retina when a series of photographs are taken.[3]

Ectopic macula

The macula may be displaced by retinal scarring or fibrous strands, often a result of retrolental fibroplasia. The displacement is usually temporal and may occur bilaterally but may also be superior or inferior and occur unilaterally after severe retinitis (*Toxocara canis*). Ectopic macula results in a displacement of the visual line and thus occasionally causes a large positive angle kappa that simulates exotropia. Congenital displacement of the macula may also occur.

Figure 23
A The Hirschberg test showed an XT of 20° to 25°.
B No shift of OD occurs when OS is covered.
C Fundus photographs reveal an ectopic macula. The tip of the fixation target (**x**) indicates the position of the fovea, which is displaced several disc diameters temporally. The retinal blood vessels are pulled over temporally. This patient had been born prematurely and for several weeks was kept in an incubator with high oxygen concentration.

34

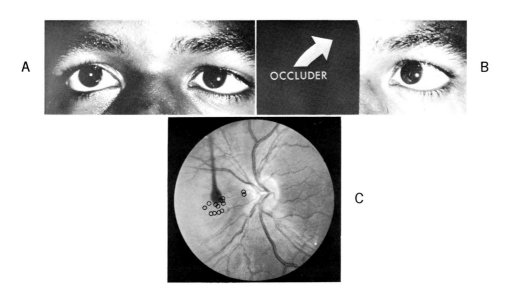

A   B

C

Figure 22

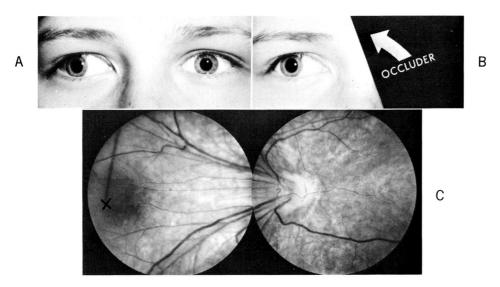

A   B

C

Figure 23

35

III. Qualitative diagnosis of strabismus

Inspection of the patient is not always sufficient for diagnosis of a manifest ocular deviation. More accurate is the following simple test.

COVER TEST FOR DETECTION OF HETEROTROPIAS

Principle: In orthophoria each eye is aligned with the fixation object. Therefore, covering of either eye will not elicit a fixation movement of the fellow eye. In heterotropia one eye is not aligned with the fixation object. Therefore, covering of the fixating eye will require the deviating eye to take up fixation, and a rapid fixation movement will result. When the deviating eye is covered, there is no movement of the fixating eye, since this eye is already aligned with the fixation object. Consequently, each eye must be covered in turn, while the fellow eye is observed to determine whether or not a heterotropia is present.

Prerequisite: Ability of the patient to fixate on an object while the test is performed.

Disadvantages: Deviation of less than 1° may escape detection with this test.[4] Small-angle strabismus with eccentric fixation cannot be diagnosed in this manner, since the amblyopic eye may fail to perform a detectable fixation movement when the sound eye is covered.

Figure 24

A Position of patient's eyes prior to the test.

B Cover placed over OS from the left does not elicit a fixation movement of OD. **No deviation of OD is present.**

C Cover placed over OD from the right does not elicit a fixation movement of OS. **No deviation of OS is present.**

D OD moves outward to fixate when OS is covered. **Esotropia.**

E OD moves inward to fixate when OS is covered. **Exotropia.**

F OD moves downward when OS is covered. **Right hypertropia.**

G OD moves upward when OS is covered. **Right hypotropia.**

When there is no fixation movement of the right eye upon covering of the left eye, the right eye has to be covered in order to exclude a manifest strabismus of the left eye.

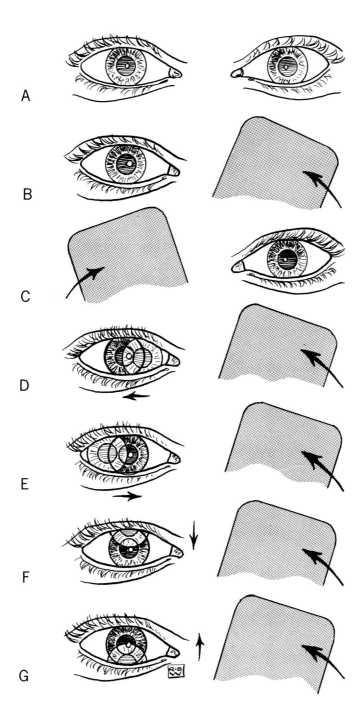

A

B

C

D

E

F

G

Figure 24

39

COVER TEST FOR DETECTION OF HETEROTROPIAS—cont'd

Indirect cover test

Figure 25

Infants and young children may object to having an occluder or the examiner's hand held directly on their face and become uncooperative. Under such circumstances the test is performed by placing the occluder at some distance between the patient's eye and the fixation object.

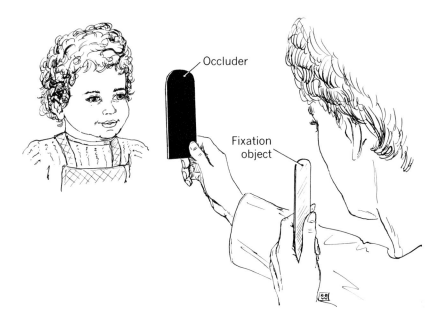

Occluder

Fixation
object

Figure 25

41

COVER-UNCOVER TEST FOR DETECTION OF HETEROPHORIAS

Principle: The monocular cover-uncover test detects deviations that are kept under control by the fusion mechanism as long as both eyes are open. However, when fusion is disrupted by covering one eye, a deviation of the covered eye occurs if a heterophoria is present. As in the cover test, each eye is covered in turn; but in this procedure the occluder is quickly removed, and the examiner notes whether or not the eye under the cover has deviated and performs a fusional movement upon removal of the cover. Occasionally, a heterophoria becomes manifest by covering either eye. It is therefore recommended that the cover test be repeated after the cover-uncover test has been performed. Heterophorias that are easily converted into heterotropias by covering one eye are characterized by weak and often insufficient fusional power. This observation is of clinical importance.

Prerequisite: Same as for cover test.

Disadvantage: Small phorias may be overlooked, but these can be detected with the Maddox rod test (Figures 31 and 32). The cover-uncover test is crude and should be employed only for screening. For quantitative determination of heterophorias, see Maddox rod test.

Figure 26

A Cover has been removed from OD, and no movement of OD can be detected. **No latent deviation of OD.**

B Cover has been removed from OS, and no movement of OS can be detected. **No latent deviation of OS.**

(If conditions in **A** and **B** are present, the patient has no phorias that can be detected with this test.)

C When uncovered, OS moves outward to fixate. **Esophoria.**

D When uncovered, OS moves inward to fixate. **Exophoria.**

E When uncovered, OS moves down to fixate. **Left hyperphoria.**

F When uncovered, OS moves up to fixate. **Left hypophoria.**

The cover-uncover test has to be performed on both eyes.

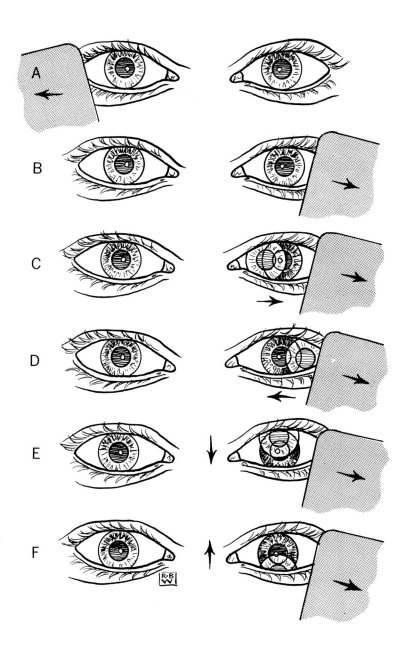

Figure 26

43

IV. Quantitative diagnosis of strabismus

HIRSCHBERG TEST

Principle: The deviation of the corneal light reflex from the center of the pupil is estimated. With the fixation light held 33 cm. from the patient, 1 mm. decentration corresponds to 7° of ocular deviation.

Procedure: A fixation light is held at eye level 33 cm. from the patient.

Prerequisites: Attention, useful visual acuity, ability to fixate on a light, and central fixation OU.

Disadvantages: Not precise. Deviations up to 7° may be overlooked. A large angle kappa may be misleading (page 32).

Figure 27

A Corneal light reflexes are in a normal position of slight nasal decentration (physiologic "positive angle kappa"; see Figure 21).

B Light reflex is at the temporal pupillary border OS. 15° esotropia.

C 30° esotropia.

D 45° esotropia.

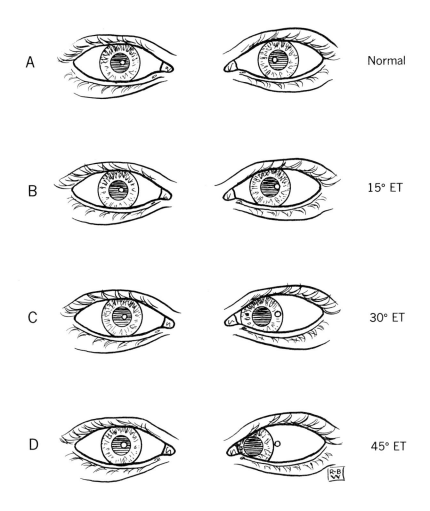

A   Normal

B   15° ET

C   30° ET

D   45° ET

Figure 27

PRISM REFLEX TEST

Principle: Prisms of increasing power are placed before the fixating eye until the light reflex is centered in the deviating eye. The prism with sufficient power to achieve centration of the light reflex indicates the magnitude of the deviation. The examiner must sit directly in front of the deviating eye in order to avoid false readings caused by parallax.

Prerequisites: Attention and ability to fixate on a light with the dominant eye.

Advantages: The test does not depend on the fixation behavior of the deviated eye, and it provides an estimate of the deviation in patients with eccentric fixation.

Disadvantage: Not precise.

Figure 28

A to **C**   Prisms, base out, of increasing power are placed before the fixating eye until the light reflex is centered on the cornea of the deviating eye (**C**).

D   Optical principles of the prism reflex test.

Remarks: The test is performed differently by many ophthalmologists. They hold the prism before the deviating eye and observe the light reflex under the prism. We find that observation of the cornea under the prism is often difficult for optical reasons and therefore prefer the procedure previously described, which is based on Hering's law of equal innervation (page 20).

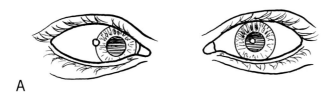

A

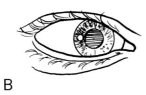

B

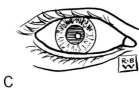

C

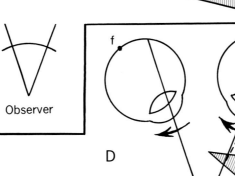

Observer

D

Figure 28

47

PRISM-COVER TEST

Principle: The cover is placed alternately over each eye. This is repeated several times to dissociate the eyes and to bring out the maximal deviation (*alternate cover test*). In order to completely dissociate the eyes it is essential to transfer the cover rapidly and never to permit momentary exposure of both eyes at a time. On the other hand, each eye must be covered sufficiently long (at least 2 seconds) to achieve complete dissociation of binocular reflexes.

The eye just uncovered makes a movement of redress opposite to the direction of the deviation. This movement of redress is compensated for by prisms of increasing power until it stops. The power of the prism is read and is equivalent to the deviation. This test must be carried out with each eye fixating in turn (to determine the primary and secondary angles of squint) at 33 cm. and at 6 m., with and without glasses. (See Figures 14 and 85.)

The influence of accommodation must be controlled by having the patient read 20/30 letters or describe a small picture while the deviation is measured at near. In exodeviations it is advisable to repeat the measurement through plus and minus 3.00 spherical lenses in order to determine the effect of accommodative convergence.

Prerequisites: Foveal fixation OU, sufficient vision to see the fixation target, and attention and cooperation sufficient to fixate on the target.

Advantages: This is a quick but gross test for the measurement of heterotropias and heterophorias. No subjective factors other than attention and cooperation are required, and the participation of the patient is limited to a minimum.

Disadvantage: Increasingly inaccurate in large deviations.

Figure 29
A Right esotropia.
B When OS is covered, OD moves outward to take over fixation.
C When the cover is transferred to OD, OS moves out to take over fixation.
D Prism, base out, is held before OD; the cover is transferred to OS. There is still outward movement of OD when taking over fixation, although the amplitude of this movement has been decreased by the effect of the prism (compare with **B**).
E The cover is again transferred, and a prism of greater power is held before OD.
F Transfer of cover to OS does not elicit fixation movement of OD; the deviation is offset by the prism, and the power of this prism equals the deviation.

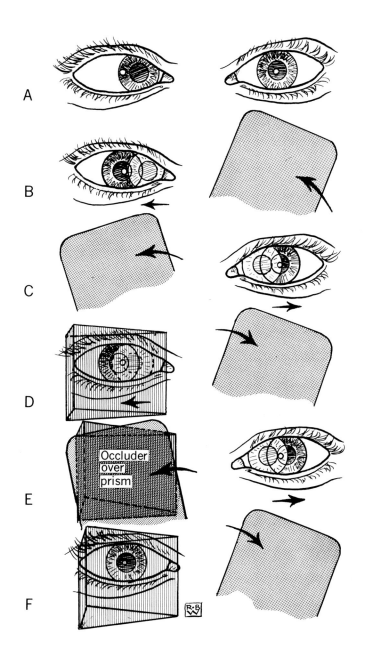

A

B

C

D

E

Occluder over prism

F

Figure 29

Figure 30. Optical principles of prism-cover test.

A Image of object fixated by OD is projected on the nasal half of the retina of OS.

B When OD is covered, OS moves outward to take over fixation. Under the cover, OD performs a movement of equal amplitude in the same direction, following Hering's law of equal innervation.

C When a prism of sufficient power offsets the nasal displacement of the image, OS will not longer change its position when OD is covered (compare with Figure 29, **F**).

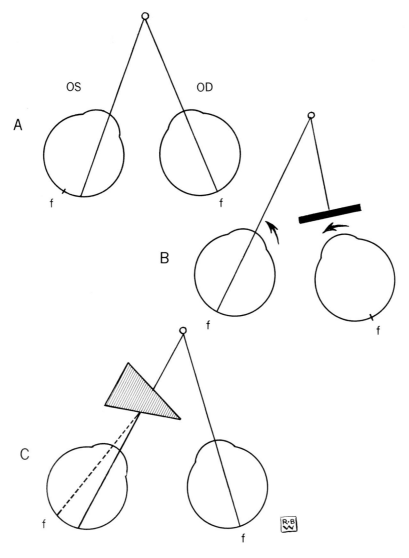

OS

OD

A

f

f

B

f

f

C

f

f

Figure 30

MADDOX ROD TEST FOR HETEROPHORIA

Principle: The eyes are dissociated by distorting one image. The Maddox rod is aligned horizontally (or vertically) before the right eye. A bright light is viewed in a darkened room with both eyes. The cylindric effect of the Maddox rod will convert the light into a vertical (or horizontal) line for the right eye. The patient indicates where he sees the light in regard to the line. Loose prisms (or a rotary prism) are superimposed on the Maddox rod until the line is centered on the light. When this has occurred, the prism power equals the amount of phoria. The test is performed at 6 m. and at 33 cm. For testing at near, the eyes must be in a reading position, a fact that is neglected in the design of all phoropters. During the test the patient must wear his spectacle correction.

Prerequisite: Vision must be sufficient to see the light with one eye and the line with the other eye.

Disadvantage: Does not differentiate between heterophorias and heterotropias. A manifest strabismus must be excluded by the cover test before the Maddox rod test is employed to measure heterophorias.

Horizontal phoria

Figure 31

A Maddox rod in testing position for horizontal heterophoria.

B Patient sees line going through light. No horizontal phoria is present.

C Line is seen to left of light (crossed diplopia). Exophoria. Add prisms, base in, to OD until line is centered on light. The power of the prism is read and equals the amount of phoria.

D Line is seen to right of light (uncrossed diplopia). Esophoria. Add prisms, base out, to OD until line is centered.

Vertical phoria

Figure 32

A Maddox rod in testing position for vertical phoria.

B No vertical phoria is present.

C Right hypophoria (usually left hyperphoria also). Add prisms, base down, to OS until line is centered.

D Right hyperphoria. Add prisms, base up, to OS until line is centered.

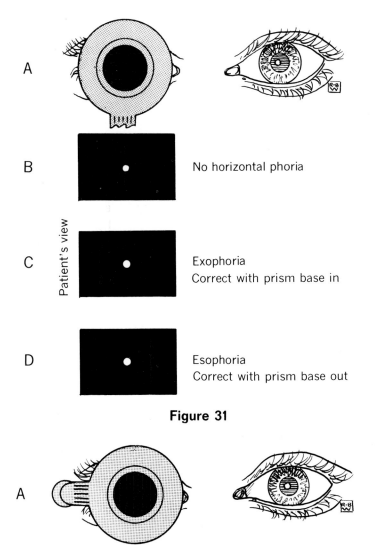

A

B   No horizontal phoria

C   Exophoria
           Correct with prism base in

D   Esophoria
           Correct with prism base out

Patient's view

Figure 31

A

B   No vertical phoria

C   Right hypophoria
           Correct with prism base
           down before OS

D   Right hyperphoria
           Correct with prism base
           up before OS

Patient's view

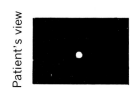

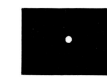

Figure 32

53

PRISM DISSOCIATION TEST

Another method for the measurement of heterophorias that is frequently used is the prism dissociation test. A 6^Δ prism, base down, is held before one eye and a rotary prism before the other. In presence of a horizontal heterophoria the patient will have vertical and horizontal diplopia. By means of the rotary prism the images are horizontally aligned until one is seen on the top of the other. The power of the prism that causes horizontal alignment indicates the size of the heterophoria.

MADDOX DOUBLE-PRISM TEST FOR CYCLODEVIATIONS

Principle: Two 4^Δ prisms are mounted together, base to base, in a frame. If the separation line between the two prisms bisects the visual axis of the patient, he will see two lines displaced vertically in opposite directions when viewing, for instance, a black horizontal line. A third line seen by the fellow eye (without a prism) will appear between the two lines. The patient judges whether or not the center line is parallel to the other lines.

Advantage: Can be done with normal room illumination, thus requiring no special light source.

Disadvantages: Permits only qualitative, not quantitative, diagnosis and does not differentiate between cyclotropia and cyclophoria. For quantitative measurements use Maddox double-rod test or Bagolini striated glasses (Figures 34 and 56).

Figure 33
A The patient views a horizontal pencil line, drawn on a white sheet of paper, with the eye to be tested (OD). The double prism is placed before the other eye (OS).
B The central line is seen by OD; the upper and lower lines, by OS. In absence of a cyclodeviation, all three lines are seen as parallel.
C The central line is tilted outward. Incyclophoria (or incyclotropia) OD.
D The central line is tilted inward. Excyclophoria (or excyclotropia) OD.

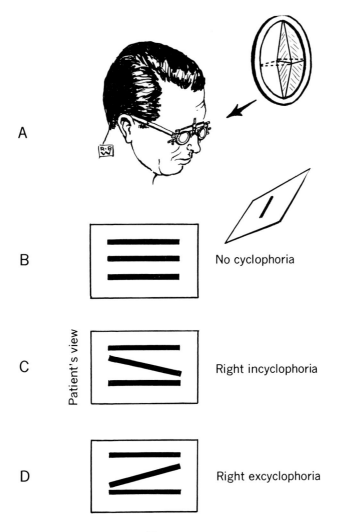

A

B   No cyclophoria

Patient's view

C   Right incyclophoria

D   Right excyclophoria

Figure 33

MADDOX DOUBLE-ROD TEST FOR CYCLODEVIATIONS

Principle: A red and a white Maddox rod are inserted into the trial frame, the red one before the eye that is suspected of having a cyclodeviation. Special care must be taken to align the direction of the glass rods with the 90° mark of the trial frame. A small scratch on the metal frame of the Maddox rod facilitates the alignment. The trial frame must be adjusted carefully to assure its exact horizontal position; the patient's head should be straight and preferably fixed. If no vertical deviation is present, a 6^Δ prism, base down, is placed before one eye, to separate the two horizontal lines seen by the patient, and thus facilitate their identification.

Advantage: Permits quantitative determination of cyclodeviations.

Disadvantages: Differentiation between cyclophoria and cyclotropia is not possible. The room must be dark.

Figure 34

A Positioning of Maddox rods in trial frame to test patient who has possible paralysis of the RSO and in whom cyclotropia of OD is suspected. Patient sees the red image intorted. This indicates excyclotropia of OD, caused in this patient by overaction of the antagonistic inferior oblique muscle.

B The Maddox rod is turned by the examiner (an intelligent patient can do it by himself) until the two lines are parallel. When parallelism has been achieved, the magnitude of cyclotropia can be read off the trial frame (7°), and the direction of the deviation is indicated by the displacement of the scratch mark on the Maddox rod from the 90° mark on the trial frame. (Here, the Maddox rod had to be rotated **out**ward to achieve parallel lines, indicating **ex**cyclotropia.)

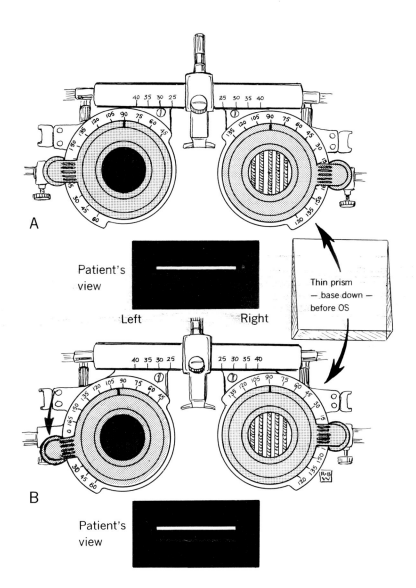

A

Patient's view

Left Right

Thin prism
— base down —
before OS

B

Patient's view

Figure 34

57

DIPLOPIA TEST FOR MEASUREMENT OF OCULAR DEVIATIONS

Principle: A dark red glass is placed before one eye. If vision is unequal, the glass should be placed before the better eye to avoid suppression of the weaker eye. It is most important that the red filter be dark enough so that the patient sees only the central fixation light of the Maddox scale. If the filter is not sufficiently dark, the patient will see two images of the Maddox scale and be unable to make exact judgments as to the position of each image.

The principle of this test is based on stimulation of both foveas, with images originating from different visual objects. The red light and the number on the Maddox scale will be localized in a common visual direction, provided retinal correspondence is normal.

Advantage: Exact determination of angle of deviation.

Disadvantages: Full cooperation of patient is required. The test is not applicable with young children. If employed in patients with ARC, the dissociating character of the test may induce an artifact and thus influence the result. It does not differentiate between heterotropia and heterophoria since dissociation of eyes may result in a heterophoria becoming a manifest deviation.

Figure 35

A The test is performed at a distance of 5 m. It can also be performed at 1 m., in which case the smaller numbers on the Maddox scale (not contained in this drawing) indicate the angle of separation. This patient has a right esotropia of 4°.

B Provided both foveas have a common visual direction (NRC), the red light will appear in the same visual direction as the number whose image is formed on the fovea of the deviating eye; in this case the light appears on number 4. If, because of suppression or ARC, the patient is unaware of the red image, a vertical prism of $6^\triangle$ to $10^\triangle$ is added base down to the red filter. Accordingly, the red image will be seen vertically displaced* (not shown in this figure).

C Homonymous diplopia in an esotropic (or esophoric) patient with 4° deviation.

---

*Both eyes are viewed from behind the orbit in this and all subsequent diagrams of this type.

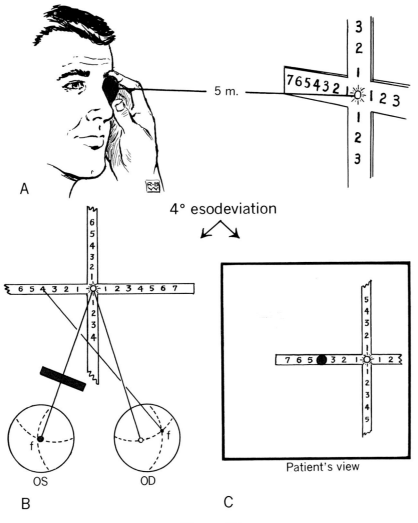

4° esodeviation

Patient's view

B   C

Figure 35

UNILATERAL VS. ALTERNATING STRABISMUS

Differentiation between these two forms is an important diagnostic step during the examination and provides instant and valuable information regarding the nature of a deviation.

If there is a strong preference for fixation with one eye (unilateral strabismus), amblyopia must immediately be suspected in the fellow eye (see also Figure 38). In infants too young to cooperate in using the illiterate "E" test, this information on preference may alone suffice to start therapy. A strong preference for fixation with one eye occurs only occasionally without amblyopia.

If the strabismus is alternating, vision is usually normal in both eyes and amblyopia is not present.

Unilateral strabismus

Figure 36
A Patient with right esotropia.
B Covering of OS requires patient to fixate with OD.
C Removal of cover results in an immediate return to fixation of OS and deviation of OD.

Conclusions: This patient has a strong preference for fixation with the left eye. Amblyopia must be suspected in the right eye. This suspicion is increased when the right eye performs searching movements or fixates unsteadily when the left eye is covered.

Alternating strabismus

Figure 37
A Patient with right esotropia.
B Covering of OS requires patient to fixate with OD; under the cover, OS turns inward.
C On uncovering of OS, OD maintains fixation and OS stays turned inward.

Conclusions: Fixation can be held with either eye, although there may still be some preference for fixation with one particular eye. It is unlikely that amblyopia is present.

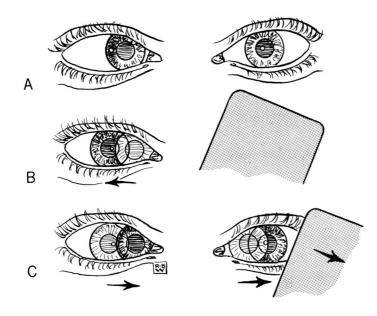

Figure 36

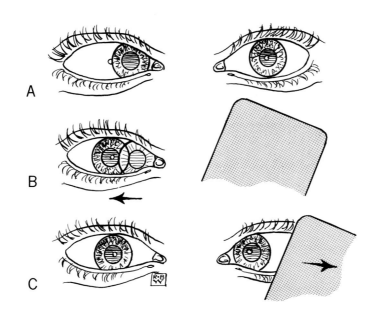

Figure 37

61

V. Evaluation of sensory state

VISUAL ACUITY

Estimation of visual acuity in infants

It is not necessary to wait until the child is old enough to play the "E" game to diagnose, treat, and (in most instances) cure amblyopia. Every child with a unilateral deviation should be suspected of amblyopia. A very simple test is available for screening even children under 1 year of age for amblyopia.

Principle: If visual acuity is equal or nearly equal in the two eyes, a child will not object to having either eye occluded. If visual acuity is reduced in one eye, the child will often cry or push the occluder aside when the sound eye is covered. If this occurs, a unilateral refractive error, fundus pathology, or amblyopia should be suspected. Once optical or organic factors have been excluded by refraction and fundus examination, amblyopia should be treated without delay by occlusion of the dominant eye until the child alternates in using his eyes. With infants this can often be achieved in 2 to 3 weeks. The cover test must be repeated at least every 2 weeks in children under the age of 4 years in order to detect and prevent the development of *occlusion amblyopia* in the formerly fixating eye.

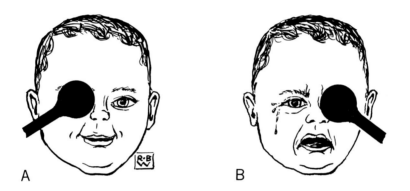

Figure 38

A child with right esotropia may not object to having the deviated eye covered (**A**), but he protests occlusion of the dominant eye (**B**). Here, amblyopia of OD must be suspected especially when the eye now performs searching or nystagmoid movements.

VISUAL ACUITY—cont'd

Determination of visual acuity in illiterate children using single optotypes and linear chart

Visual acuity can be determined once the child has reached the age of 2½ to 3 years and is sufficiently cooperative to perform the "E" game. The mother is instructed to teach the child this test at home, beginning at near vision and with both eyes open and slowly increasing the test distance. The child is taught to indicate with his hand or with a large test letter the direction in which the three bars of the test letter held by the examiner are pointing (Figure 39, A). Once the child comprehends the test and visual acuity has been determined by finding the smallest optotype read with each eye at 20 feet, the test is repeated, exposing each time one line of the illiterate chart. It may be necessary to point to the letter to be identified (Figure 39, B): Exposing the optotypes in a linear arrangement will frequently permit detection of amblyopia in children who show normal vision with isolated letters (crowding phenomenon).

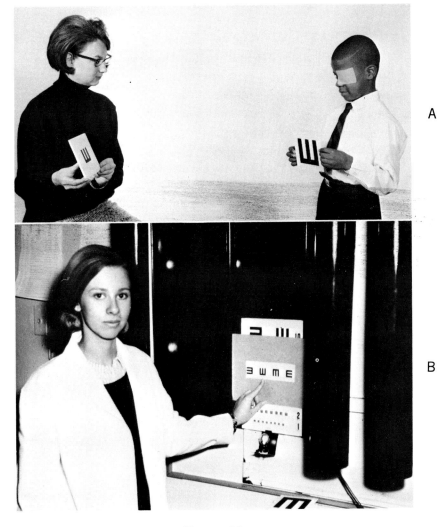

Figure 39

65

SUPPRESSION
Worth four-dot test

Principle: A red glass filters out all colors except red. Thus a green light will be invisible through a red filter; vice versa, every color except green will become invisible when viewed through a green filter.

Prerequisites: Absence of deep amblyopia. Sufficient patient cooperation is necessary, since interpretation depends on subjective responses.

Disadvantages: This is a very gross test. Even in the presence of dense central suppression scotomas or of small-angle deviations, the results may indicate "fusion." The test provides information only about the status of peripheral binocular cooperation.

Figure 40

A Looking through a pair of red and green goggles, the patient views a box with four lights (one red, two green, and one white) at 6 m. and at 33 cm. (with the four lights mounted on a flashlight). The possible responses are given in **B** to **E**.

B Patient sees all four lights: peripheral fusion with orthophoria or a small-angle esotropia with ARC.

C Patient sees two vertically displaced red lights: suppression OS.

D Patient sees three green lights: suppression OD.

E Patient sees five lights. The red lights may appear to the right, as in this figure (uncrossed diplopia with esotropia), or to the left of the green lights (crossed diplopia with exotropia).

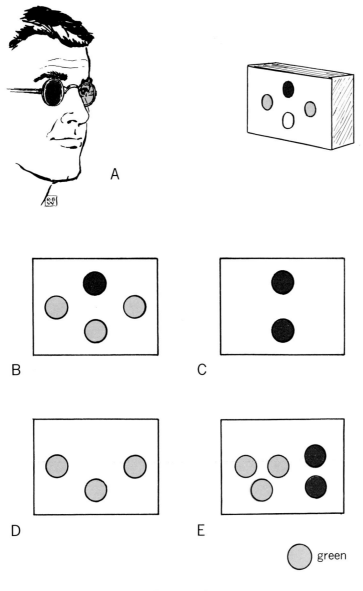

A

B

C

D

E

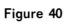 green

Figure 40

SUPPRESSION—cont'd

4△ base-out prism test

Principle: Small central suppression scotomas (1° to 2°) in patients with very small angles of esotropia, with microstrabismus (Figures 51 to 53), or with previous surgical correction of a larger deviation are difficult to detect. Image displacement, by using a weak base-out prism and observing the resulting binocular (version) and monocular (fusional) eye movements, is a quick and sensitive screening procedure to assess whether or not bifoveal fusion or suppression of one fovea is present. Sudden displacement of an image (by means of a prism, base out) from one fovea onto the parafoveal temporal retina will elicit a refixation movement if the image has been shifted within a normally functioning retina, but no movement will occur if the image has been shifted within a nonfunctioning (that is, within a scotomatous) area. According to Hering's law, the movement of the fellow eye will be biphasic: this eye will move outward simultaneously and symmetrically (version) when the eye under the prism refixates; and it subsequently performs a slow fusional movement (duction) in the opposite direction to correct for the image displacement. However, if a central scotoma has impaired foveal function, the second phase, the fusional movement, does not occur and the eye remains slightly turned out.

Advantage: Cooperation of the patient is limited to his attention and ability to hold fixation during the test.

Disadvantages: Several atypical responses are possible that limit the usefulness of this test as a screening device.[5] In patients with deficient fusional convergence but otherwise normal binocular functions the characteristic biphasic movement of the eye without the prism may be absent.

Procedure: A 4△ base-out prism is quickly placed over the right eye while the patient fixates on a point light source and the examiner observes the movements of the left eye. The test is repeated by placing the prism over the left eye and observing the right eye.

Figure 41

A On placing the prism over OD, levoversion occurs during refixation of OD. This indicates absence of foveal suppression OD.

B A subsequent slow fusional movement of OS is observed to correct for the image displacement. This indicates absence of foveal suppression OS.

C In another patient, OS remains abducted 4△ after a prism is placed over OD. Absence of the secondary fusional movement of OS indicates a foveal suppression scotoma of OS. The image has been shifted within a nonfunctioning retinal area. No stimulus exists for refusion.

D To confirm this diagnosis the prism is placed over OS. Neither eye will move under these circumstances, since the prism has merely displaced the image within the suppression scotoma and no stimulus exists for refixation.

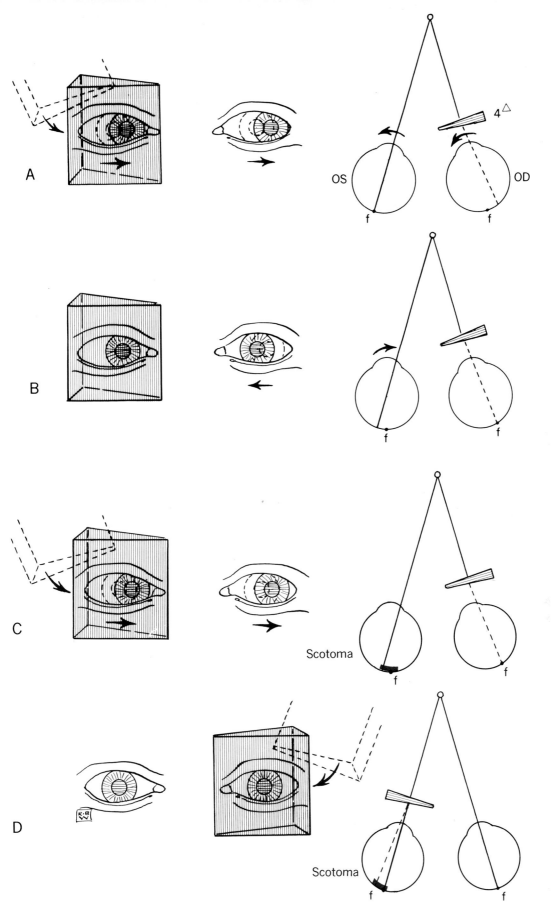

Figure 41

69

SUPPRESSION—cont'd

Red glass test for suppression and retinal correspondence

Principle: If a patient with heterotropia reports no diplopia, he may be suppressing or ignoring the second image visible in the periphery of the field of vision. Holding a red glass over the fixating eye while the patient is viewing a bright light will draw his attention to the second (white) image if it has been ignored. Only the red light will be seen if deep suppression or ARC is present. The test can also be used to identify a paretic muscle by measuring the distance between the two images in the diagnostic positions of gaze (muscle fields).

The depth of suppression can be quantitated by increasing the density of the filter held before the fixating eye until the patient reports diplopia.

Figure 42

A Fixation light is viewed with a red filter held before the fixating left eye. Uncrossed diplopia with esotropia. The white light stimulates nasal retina of OD and is localized to the right.

B Crossed diplopia in exotropia. The white light stimulates temporal retina of OD and is localized to the left.

C Image formed by the fixation light falls on a suppression scotoma in the right eye of an esotropic patient and is not seen. Suppression or ARC may be present. If under these circumstances a **dark** red filter is placed before the fixating eye, diplopia can be elicited even in the presence of deep suppression.

D In order to differentiate between suppression and ARC a prism, base up, is held before the deviated eye, displacing the image upward and beyond the suppression area. With NRC the light will appear below and to the right; with ARC it will appear horizontally aligned with, but vertically separated from, the red light.

70

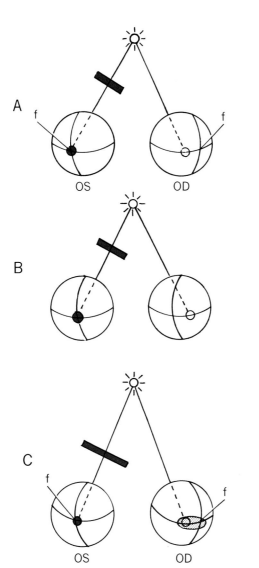

A

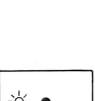

Patient's view

B

C

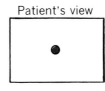

Patient's view

D

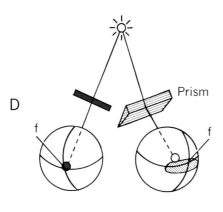

Prism

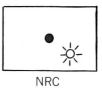

NRC

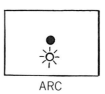

ARC

Figure 42

71

SUPPRESSION—cont'd

Measurement of size of suppression scotoma

The size of the suppression scotoma is most accurately determined by binocular perimetry. A less accurate but nevertheless useful clinical method consists of mapping out the size of the scotoma by prism-induced image displacement.

Procedure: A rotary prism is held before the patient's deviated eye. Base-out power is increased until the patient reports diplopia. At that point the image has left the temporal border of the scotoma. The nasal border of the scotoma is determined by prisms base-in until diplopia occurs. The vertical borders of the scotoma are defined in a similar manner with vertical prisms. A light red filter before the fixating eye facilitates recognition of diplopia by the patient.

Figure 43

A In right esotropia the image of the visual object fixated by the left eye falls on nasal retinal elements of the deviated right eye. Suppression eliminates diplopia.

B Base-out prisms before OD are increased until crossed diplopia occurs; the temporal border of the scotoma has been defined.

C Base-in prisms before OD are increased until uncrossed diplopia occurs; the nasal border of the scotoma has been defined. The total prismatic power required to move the image from the temporal to the nasal border of the scotoma indicates its horizontal diameter.

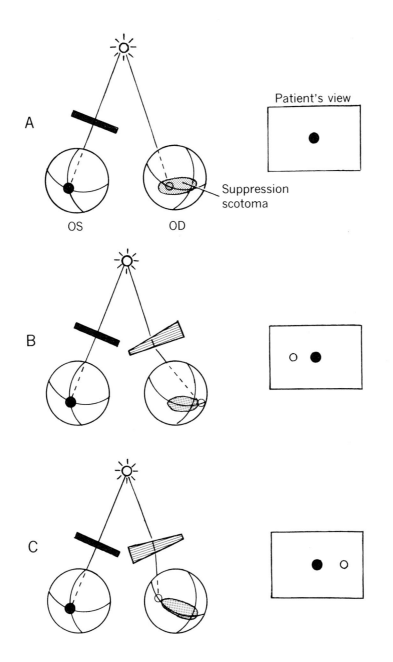

Patient's view

Suppression
scotoma

OS   OD

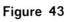

Figure 43

73

SUPPRESSION—cont'd

Blind-spot syndrome

Patients with persistent esotropia of 25^Δ to 35^Δ at distance and at near fixation may utilize the blind spot of the deviated eye in order to avoid diplopia in binocular vision.[6] The image in the deviated eye falls on the optic nerve head. Monocularly, visual acuity of the deviated eye is usually normal; fusion may be demonstrated, with the angle of deviation corrected by a major amblyoscope. Occasional diplopia may occur when the image falls on the peripapillary retina, and confusion of foveal images (Figure 45, *A*) may be present.

Figure 44

A Blind-spot syndrome in an esotropic patient. The image falls on the optic disc of the deviated right eye. The patient experiences single vision but may have confusion of different images unless foveal suppression is present, since an object different from that fixated by OS falls on the fovea of the deviated eye.

B For diagnostic purposes the deviation is reduced by a base-out prism. The image is now formed between the optic disc and the fovea of the right eye. The patient experiences uncrossed diplopia.

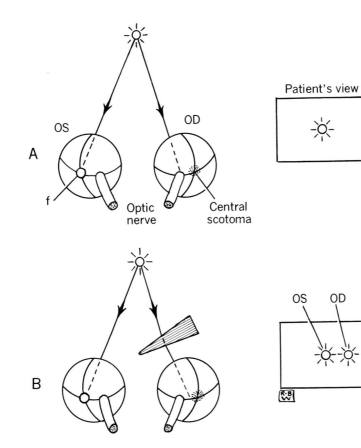

A

Patient's view

OS

OD

f

Optic
nerve

Central
scotoma

B

OS   OD

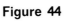

Figure 44

AMBLYOPIA

Mechanism of amblyopia

The following conditions may lead to an impairment of foveal vision that is partially or totally reversible by appropriate therapy.

Figure 45

A **Strabismus.** In a patient with right esotropia the fovea of OD (f) is aligned with a different visual object "Δ" than the visual object fixated foveally by OS, "O." Since the images formed on the fovea of each eye are localized in a common visual direction, the patient will see two different visual objects superimposed in subjective space (**"confusion"**). Also, the image of the object "O" will be formed on nasal retinal elements (e) of OD and thus be localized in the temporal field of vision (diplopia). **Confusion** and **diplopia** (if present in children under 7 years of age) may cause suppression of the fovea and of peripheral retinal elements (nasal retina in esotropia, temporal retina in exotropia). When suppression persists on covering of the fixating eye, amblyopia is present.

B **Anisometropia.** When the foveal images in the two eyes are of different size and shape because of unequal refraction, an obstacle to fusion is present. Small differences are tolerated. Larger differences in refraction (more than 2.5 D between the two eyes) may disturb binocular function, although some patients tolerate even larger image-size differences without complaints. Some patients develop alternating vision (using the more myopic eye for near vision and the fellow eye for distance vision), or they suppress the blurred image of one eye. This may lead to amblyopia (anisometropic amblyopia).

C **Organic factors.** Damage (usually of unknown cause) to the visual system, anywhere between the retina and the striate cortex, may reduce foveal function in one eye and cause a relative or an absolute scotoma without ophthalmoscopic findings. The resulting blurred foveal image may interfere with fusion. If this occurs, a functional (reversible) suppression scotoma may become superimposed on the organic (irreversible) visual impairment (**relative amblyopia**). Strabismus may develop secondary to decreased foveal function (sensory strabismus).

D **Form vision deprivation (amblyopia ex anopsia).** Opacities of the ocular media (corneal clouding, cataract) may interfere with the formation of a well-focused image on the fovea; only diffuse light can enter the eye. In children up to the age of 5 years this may cause amblyopia. Usually, this form of amblyopia is irreversible and severe; it may occur in one or both eyes.[7] A milder and often reversible form occurs after prolonged occlusion in the formerly dominant eye of a strabismic child (**occlusion amblyopia**).

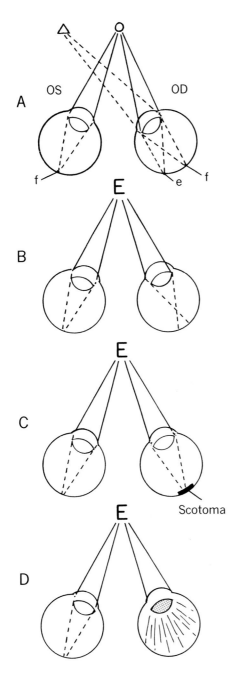

A

OS   OD

f   e   f

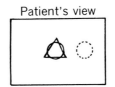

Patient's view

B

E

C

E

Scotoma

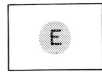

D

E

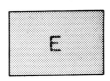

Figure 45

AMBLYOPIA—cont'd

Neutral density filter test

This test is employed prior to occlusion or pleoptic treatment to differentiate between functional and organic amblyopia. A combination of neutral density filters (Kodak No. 96; N.D. 2.00 and 0.50) of sufficient density to reduce visual acuity in normal eyes from 20/20 to 20/40 is placed before the amblyopic eye. This will reduce acuity by one or two lines, leave it unaffected, or even cause a slight improvement of vision if the impairment is functional (reversible) in nature. When organic amblyopia is present, visual acuity is often markedly reduced by the filter.[8]

Advantage: Allows quick screening in the office before proceeding with occlusion therapy in amblyopias of uncertain origin.

Disadvantage: Test is difficult to quantitate in patients with deep amblyopia (less than 20/200).

Figure 46

A While the sound eye is occluded, the filter is held before the amblyopic eye for 1 minute before visual acuity is determined.

B Without the filter the patient reads 20/40.

C With the filter, vision remains 20/40 (or it may improve one or two lines) in **functional** amblyopia.

D The filter may reduce visual acuity three or more lines in cases of **organic** amblyopia.

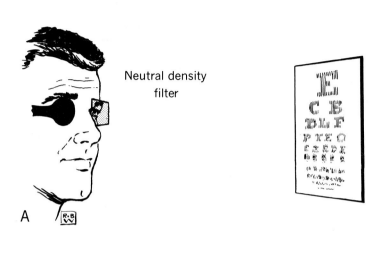

Neutral density filter

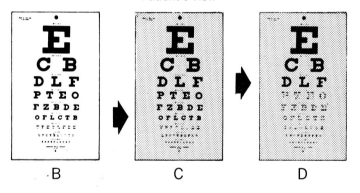

Patient's view

B   C   D

Figure 46

AMBLYOPIA—cont'd

Determination of fixation behavior

It is not sufficient to base the diagnosis of the fixation behavior on the position of the corneal light reflex. Parafoveal and paramacular fixation may escape diagnosis, and an abnormal angle kappa may simulate eccentric fixation where none is present. Fixation is diagnosed with the Visuscope and may be documented with the Zeiss fundus camera.

Visuscope:

Figure 47

The Visuscope is a modified ophthalmoscope that projects a fixation target on the fundus. The eye that is not to be tested is occluded. The examiner projects the fixation target close to the macula, and the patient is directed to look at the black asterisk. The position of the asterisk on the patient's fundus is noted. This test is repeated several times to obtain information about the size of the eccentric fixation area.[3]

Fixation photography:

Serial fundus photographs are taken while the patient looks directly at the tip of the fixation target incorporated in the fundus camera.[9] This method is also employed to identify the position of the fovea before using photocoagulation or laser coagulation in the treatment of macular disease.

Figure 48

A Positions of the fixation target, documented in 18 consecutive photographs, are superimposed in this figure in order to show that this patient fixates steadily within a well-circumscribed retinal area 3° to 5° nasal to and below the fovea (VOD: 20/200).

B Summary of the different positions of the target in a patient with eccentric fixation nasal to the optic disc (VOS: 20/200). Note that the fixation area is larger than in **A.** There is a direct relationship between the size of the fixation area and its distance from the fovea.[3]

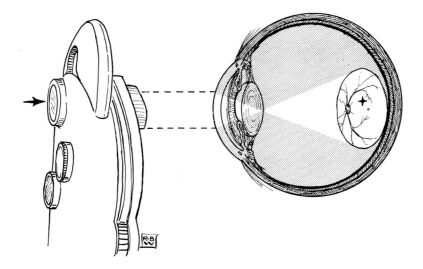

Figure 47

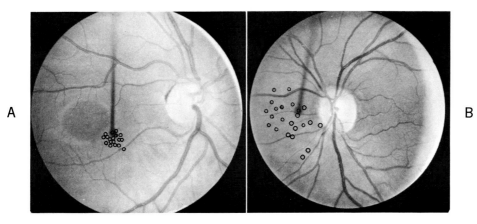

Figure 48

AMBLYOPIA—cont'd

Classification of fixation behavior

Figure 49

A Central fixation. The asterisk is fixated steadily by the fovea. In some patients small-amplitude to-and-fro oscillations of the fixated target can be observed. This micronystagmus may affect visual acuity and may occur in the absence of strabismus.

B Parafoveal eccentric fixation. The asterisk is fixated parafoveally but within the macular area.

C Paramacular eccentric fixation. Fixation occurs near the upper nasal border of the macula. Fixation becomes less steady the farther away it is from the fovea.

D Peripheral eccentric fixation. Fixation occurs outside the macula. Repeated tests frequently reveal, as shown in this drawing, that a different retinal area takes up fixation each time. By means of repeated Visuscope examinations or serial fixation photographs, it is thus possible to map out a fixation area that may measure 2 disc diameters or more in size.[3]

E Paradoxical fixation. An esotropic patient may fixate temporal to the macula, or an exotropic patient may fixate nasally. This fixation behavior is opposite from what might be expected on the basis of the ocular deviation, and such paradoxical fixation can be found after surgical overcorrection, spontaneous reversal of a deviation, after prolonged occlusion of the sound eye in amblyopia, or without any obvious cause.[10]

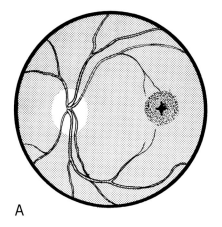

A

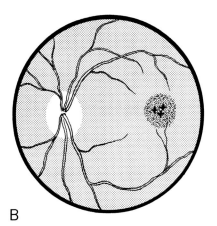

B

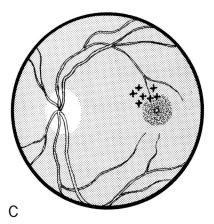

C

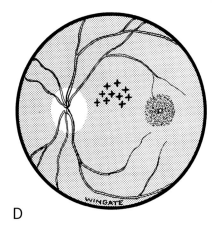

D

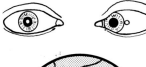

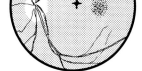

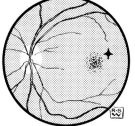

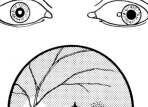

E

Figure 49

83

AMBLYOPIA—cont'd

Eccentric viewing vs. eccentric fixation

Eccentric viewing is an intermediate stage between central and eccentric fixation. In *eccentric viewing* the motor component of the fixation reflex remains oriented toward the fovea, even though foveal function is reduced. In *eccentric fixation* the fixation reflex becomes adjusted to nonfoveal (paramacular) retinal elements. Eccentric viewing occurs frequently with macular retinopathy even though eccentric fixation may gradually develop in such patients, especially when there is bilateral involvement. Clinical differentiation between eccentric viewing and eccentric fixation is more of theoretical than of practical interest.[10]

Figure 50

A In order to determine whether eccentric viewing or eccentric fixation is present in the left amblyopic eye, the examiner projects the Visuscope asterisk onto the paramacular retinal region (**1**) of the patient. The sound eye is occluded.

B The patient is requested to look directly at the asterisk (**1**) while the examiner observes the fundus through the Visuscope. First, the patient responds with an eye movement that will place the image of the fixation target on the fovea (**2**), where it is only dimly seen by the patient because of reduced foveal function (scotoma, organic lesion). Second, the eye will move in such a manner as to place the image from the fovea onto paramacular retinal element (**3**), where visual acuity in this patient may be better than in the fovea. **Eccentric viewing** is present.

C The first eye movement displaces the asterisk directly from (**1**) to (**2**), thus excluding the fovea from the act of fixation. The fixation reflex has adapted itself to paramacular nasal retinal elements. **Eccentric fixation** is present.

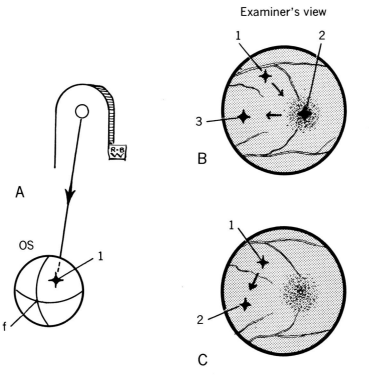

Examiner's view

A

OS

f

B

C

Figure 50

AMBLYOPIA—cont'd

Microstrabismus

Lang[11] has coined the term "microstrabismus" to describe various forms of small-angle esotropias with partial or complete sensorial adaptation. In recent years, with the introduction of more refined diagnostic techniques, it has become apparent that there exists a spectrum of anomalies of bifoveal fusion, which ranges from orthophoria or heterophoria with reduced foveal function in one eye (functional or organic scotoma) to small-angle esotropia with incomplete or complete sensorial adaptation. Parks[12] has introduced the term "monofixational syndrome" to describe the absence of bifoveal fusion in this entity.

Of the various manifestations of microstrabismus one type deserves special consideration, for it represents a uniquely complete sensorial adaptation to a minute misalignment of the eyes and poses special diagnostic problems.[13] This syndrome consists of unilateral amblyopia with parafoveal fixation, harmonious ARC, peripheral fusion with amplitudes, and up to 60% normal stereoacuity. Characteristically, the cover test is negative because on covering of the dominant eye the amblyopic eye continues to fixate with the same parafoveal retinal elements that receive the image when both eyes are open. Under binocular conditions ARC is present; the degree of eccentricity of fixation (with the dominant eye covered) equals the angle of anomaly (with both eyes open).

The incidence of this form of microstrabismus is especially high in patients with anisometropic amblyopia.

The diagnosis is based on visual acuity measurement, visuscopy, cover test, 4^Δ base-out prism test, and the bifoveal correspondence test.

The diagnostic procedures are demonstrated in Figures 51 to 53, showing microstrabismus in a 17-year-old boy with anisometropia (OD: -1.50 sph; OS $+0.50$ sph) and amblyopia (OD: 20/100).

Figure 51

A Eyes appear straight. A central suppression scotoma OD is present and has led to parafoveal fixation.

B Cover test fails to reveal a fixation movement; OD continues to fixate with the same extrafoveal elements that are used for fixation when both eyes are open.

C Visuscope reveals fixation OD 2° to 3° nasal to and slightly below the fovea.

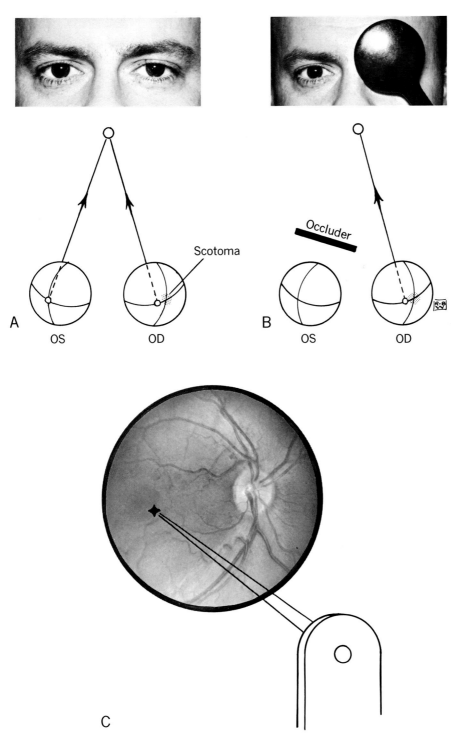

Scotoma

A

OS   OD

Occluder

B

OS   OD

C

Figure 51

87

Microstrabismus—cont'd

Figure 52

A The 4$^{\Delta}$ base-out prism test (Figure 41) does not elicit a movement of either eye when the prism is placed before OD, since the image has merely been shifted by the prism to an area within the suppression scotoma.

B When the prism is placed before OS, both eyes move to the right because OS refixates on the image (displaced temporally by the prism) and OD has to follow, according to Hering's law. However, OD fails to perform a subsequent fusional movement in the opposite direction because no fusional impulse is elicited from stimulation of retinal elements within the suppression scotoma.

Figure 53

The Bagolini test (Figure 56) reveals harmonious ARC between the fovea OS and the parafoveal retinal elements OD. The gap seen in the stripe by the amblyopic eye is caused by the foveal scotoma. The angle of anomaly can be quantitatively determined with the Cüppers test (Figure 59).

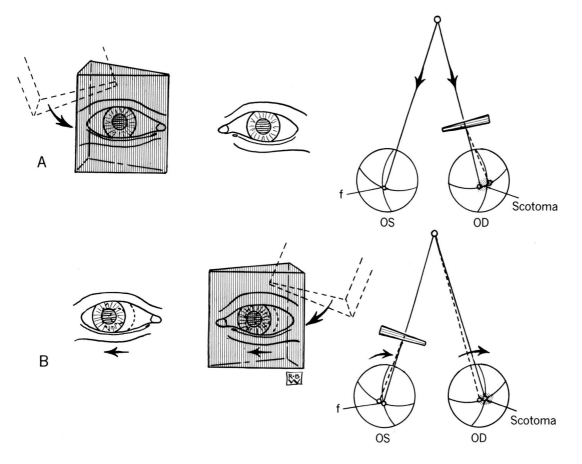

Figure 52

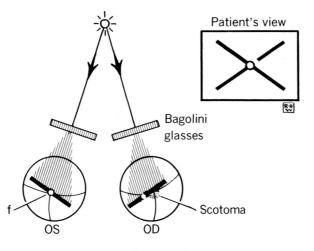

Figure 53

89

AMBLYOPIA—cont'd

Bilateral eccentric fixation

This rare anomaly occurs in congenital amblyopia of both eyes and in patients with bilateral macular disease of long duration. Under exceptional circumstances bilateral eccentric fixation occurs in a strabismic patient without evidence of macular disease.

Figure 54

A Bilateral esotropia has been present in this 18-year-old patient since the age of 1½ years.
B OD remains in an esotropic position when OS is covered.
C OS remains in an esotropic position when OD is covered.
D OD abducts well on examination of the versions.
E OS abducts well (strabismus fixus is not present).

Figure 55

A Fixation OD with an area in the nasal inferior periphery.
B Fixation OS with an area in the nasal inferior periphery.

Figures 54 and 55 from von Noorden, G. K.: Bilateral eccentric fixation, Arch. Ophthalmol. **69**:25, 1963.

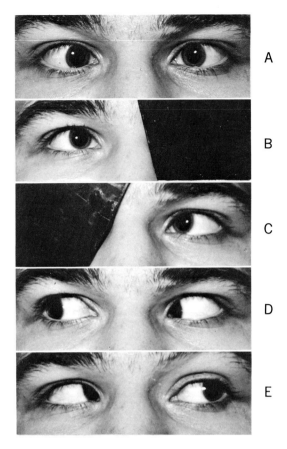

A

B

C

D

E

Figure 54

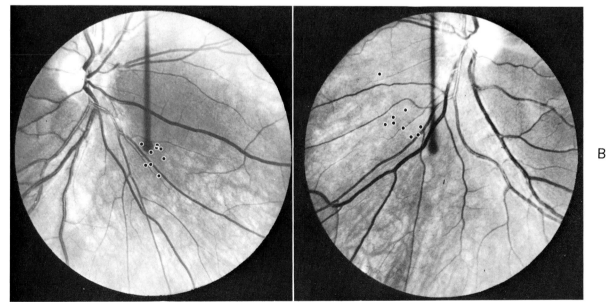

A

B

Figure 55

RETINAL CORRESPONDENCE
Bagolini striated glass test

Principle: All conventional tests for retinal correspondence introduce some degree of alteration of normal conditions of seeing. Each of the tests, by dissociating the eyes, creates an "apparatus situation" that may influence the result. An exception is the test with Bagolini glasses, which consist of optically plano lenses with imperceptible striations that hardly blur the environment but produce a luminous stripe when a person is looking at a point light source.[14] The optic principle is similar to that of the Maddox rod. The glasses are mounted in a regular spectacle frame or are placed into a trial frame before the corrective lenses. A small mark at the margin of each glass indicates the direction of striation. The glasses should be placed before the patient's eye in such a manner that the axis of striation is oriented at 135° (OD) and 45° (OS), respectively. The test is performed at 33 cm. and at 6 m. It is advisable to eliminate all other bright light sources in the examination area during this test.

Advantages: Permits investigation of retinal correspondence under nearly normal conditions of seeing without dissociation of eyes, while the position of the eyes can be checked by the examiner with the cover test. Small suppression scotomas can be diagnosed when the patient notes a gap in the luminous stripe.

The Bagolini glasses can also be employed to measure cyclotropia under ordinary conditions of seeing. The testing arrangement is similar to that described for the Maddox double-rod test (Figure 34).

Disadvantages: Extensive suppression may interfere with perception of the second stripe.

Figure 56
A Bagolini glasses mounted or in trial frame.
B If cover test reveals no shift and fixation is central, the patient has NRC. If cover test reveals a shift, there is harmonious ARC. For interpretation of results obtained in eccentric fixation, see Figure 53.
C Foveal suppression OD with peripheral fusion. If no shift occurs with cover test, NRC exists; if shift occurs, ARC exists.
D Foveal and peripheral suppression OD.

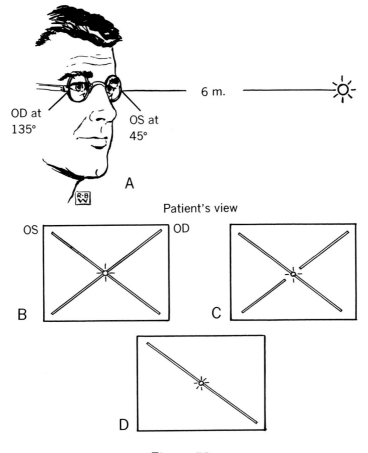

OD at
135°

OS at
45°

6 m.

A

Patient's view

OS   OD

B

C

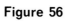

D

Figure 56

93

RETINAL CORRESPONDENCE—cont'd
Hering-Bielschowsky afterimage test

Principle: Afterimages have many characteristics of real objects and persist long after cessation of the original stimulus. Once an afterimage is created in each eye, their position in relation to each other no longer depends on whether the eyes are open, closed, straight, or crossed.

Procedure: Each eye fixates on the center black mark of a glowing filament, first presented horizontally to the eye with better visual acuity and then vertically to the poorer eye for 20 seconds in a darkened room while the fellow eye is occluded. The patient indicates the relative position of the two gaps in the center of each afterimage. The gaps correspond to the visual direction of each fovea if central fixation is present. *The interpretation of this test depends on the result of the preceding determination of the fixation behavior.*

Interpretation with central fixation:

Figure 57

A If the Visuscope examination reveals central fixation, the interpretations given in **B** to **D** are possible.

B The two foveas have a common visual direction in NRC; patient sees the gaps superimposed.

C In ARC, the two foveas no longer have a common visual direction; a patient with right ET sees the vertical afterimage displaced to the left.

D Analogous situation in right XT with ARC; vertical afterimage displaced to the right.

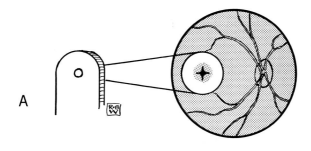

A

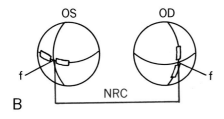

OS   OD

Patient's view

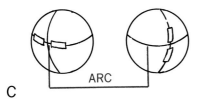

f

f

NRC

B

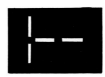

ARC

C

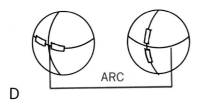

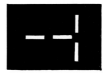

ARC

D

Figure 57

RETINAL CORRESPONDENCE—cont'd

Hering-Bielschowsky afterimage test—cont'd

Interpretation with eccentric fixation:

Figure 58

A Visuscope examination shows the asterisk to be between the fovea and disc on the nasal retina. The interpretations given in **B** and **C** are possible.

B With NRC (very rare in patients with eccentric fixation[10]), or when the angle of anomaly is not identical with the degree of eccentricity (frequent), the afterimage in the right eye will be localized uncrossed to the right.

C In small-angle strabismus the patient may employ the same extrafoveal retinal elements for fixation (the sound eye being covered) that have formed a common visual direction with the fovea of the sound eye under binocular conditions (ARC). The degree of eccentricity of fixation is then equal to the angle of anomaly (see also under discussion on micro-strabismus, page 86); **superimposition of the gaps indicates ARC** under these circumstances.

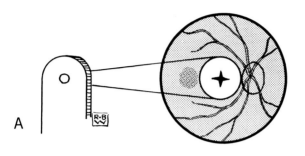

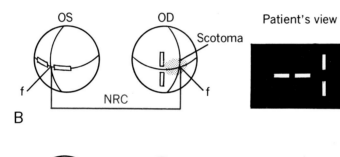

OS   OD   Patient's view

Scotoma

f   f

NRC

B

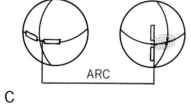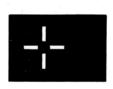

ARC

C

Figure 58

RETINAL CORRESPONDENCE—cont'd
Cüppers test for retinal correspondence

Principle: The test determines whether the two foveas have common or different visual directions. It permits quantitative analysis of the angle of anomaly when eccentric fixation is present.[15]

Advantage: This test permits determination of the angle of anomaly in the presence of eccentric fixation.

Disadvantages: The dissociating nature of this test may produce artifacts. In the presence of deep suppression the Visuscope asterisk is not seen by the amblyopic eye.

Procedure: The patient fixates with the normal eye on the central light of a Maddox scale via a plano mirror which, for the convenience of the examiner, is turned in such a manner that the amblyopic eye looks straight ahead. The Visuscope asterisk is projected by the examiner onto the fovea of the amblyopic eye. The figure of the Maddox scale on which the asterisk is seen by the patient indicates the angle of anomaly. The mirror effect has to be taken into account when the patient reports the position of the asterisk on the Maddox scale.

Figure 59

A Schematic representation of the testing arrangement. If the test is performed at 5 m. distance from the Maddox scale, the large figures indicate the angle of anomaly. The small figures (not shown in this drawing) are valid for a distance of 1 m. This patient has eccentric fixation in OD; **e** indicates the area of fixation.

B Patient sees the asterisk superimposed on the central fixation light of the Maddox scale. The two foveas have a common visual direction, indicating NRC.

C Asterisk appears over the number 4 on the horizontal bar of the Maddox scale. The two foveas have different visual directions, indicating ARC. The angle of anomaly is 4°.

Modification: In order to determine which parts of the peripheral retina in the deviating eye have acquired a common visual direction with the fovea of the fixating eye, the patient is asked to guide the Visuscope until he sees the asterisk superimposed on the central light of the Maddox cross. The examiner views the fundus when this task is completed and notes the position of the asterisk, which indicates the location of retinal elements having a common visual direction with the fovea of the sound eye.

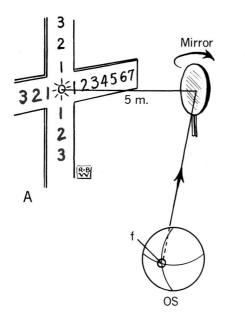

A

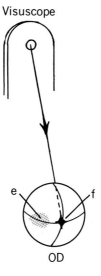

Mirror

Visuscope

OS

OD

f

e   f

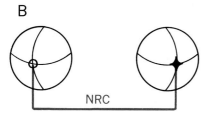

B

NRC

Patient's view

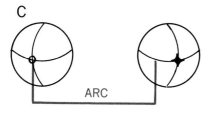

C

ARC

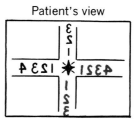

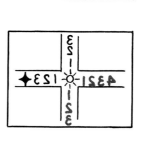

Figure 59

99

Monocular afterimage (so-called afterimage transfer) test

For the correct interpretation of this test (which is also erroneously described as the afterimage transfer test) it is absolutely essential to relate the fixation as determined by the Visuscope to the subjective response of the patient. Provided this is done, the test can be used to determine the behavior of retinal correspondence and to measure the angle of anomaly in the presence of central and eccentric fixation. It also permits one to determine the degree of eccentricity in nonfoveal fixators.

Principle: A vertical afterimage is created above and below the fovea of the fixating eye while the deviating eye is occluded (Figure 60, *A*). The occluder is switched to the fixating eye while the formerly deviating eye fixates upon the central light of a Maddox scale (Figure 60, *B*). The patient is requested to indicate the position of the vertical afterimage in relationship to the fixation light. The position of the vertical afterimage in subjective space indicates the principal visual direction of the fovea of the now occluded leading eye. The following responses may be obtained with left esotropia.

Figure 60

A Vertical afterimage is produced in OD.

B Patient views fixation light with the nonstimulated left eye and observes position of afterimage in relation to light.

C NRC in a patient with central fixation.

D ARC in a patient with eccentric fixation. The angle of anomaly corresponds to the degree of eccentricity.

E NRC in a patient with eccentric viewing.

F ARC in a patient with central fixation. The angle of anomaly corresponds to the number on the Maddox cross on which the vertical afterimage is seen.

Disadvantages: It may be difficult to make the patient aware of the afterimage when he fixates with the habitually deviated eye. Frequent blinking or flickering room illumination may enhance awareness of the afterimage. If suppression in the amblyopic eye is very deep, the afterimage is not seen at all. In such instances this test cannot be applied.

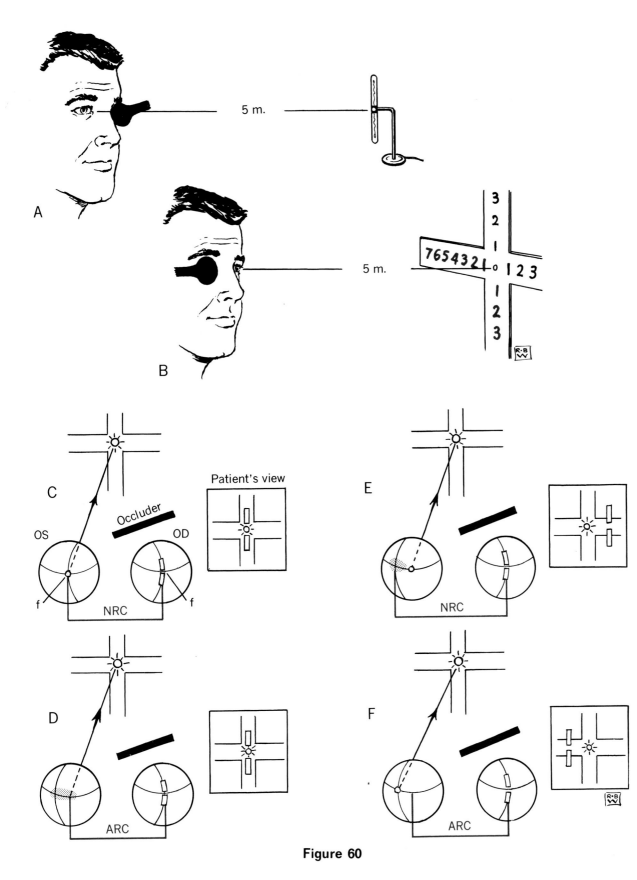

Figure 60

RETINAL CORRESPONDENCE—cont'd

Major amblyoscope

This instrument or one of its variations (troposcope, synoptophore) is indispensable for the diagnosis of anomalies of binocular vision and for orthoptic therapy. Illuminated slides with visual targets of various sizes and shapes are presented to each eye through a haploscopic arrangement. The two arms of the instrument can be moved horizontally and vertically. Diagnostic uses of the amblyoscope include the cover and alternate cover tests, the measurement of the angle of strabismus and of the degree and range of fusion, and the determination of the state of suppression and of retinal correspondence. Only the latter application will be discussed here.

Figure 61

A Both arms of the instrument are moved by the examiner while flashing the light behind each slide alternatingly until there is no further fixation movement of the patient's eye (alternate cover test). Each arm of the instrument is now set at $10^\triangle$ ET; the patient has an esotropia of $20^\triangle$. The angle of strabismus determined in this manner is called the **objective angle**. If the patient sees the visual targets superimposed when the instrument is in this position, his **subjective angle** equals the objective angle; NRC is present. When the patient reports that the targets are separated with the instrument set at the objective angle, ARC is present; his foveas no longer have a common visual direction (paradoxical diplopia, Figure 62).

B When the patient reports superimposition of the visual targets with the instrument arms set at zero, his subjective angle is zero and ARC is present. In this case the **angle of anomaly** equals the objective angle and the sensory adaptation is complete: ARC is **harmonious**.

C When the angle of anomaly is smaller than the objective angle, **unharmonious** abnormal retinal correspondence is present. In this drawing a patient with $20^\triangle$ ET reports superimposition with the arms of the instrument set at $10^\triangle$ ET. The sensory adaptation is incomplete; the subjective angle is smaller ($10^\triangle$ ET) than the objective angle ($20^\triangle$ ET), but larger than zero. In most instances unharmonious ARC can be explained on the basis of a secondary enlargement of the objective angle; some authors have suspected that this finding is an instrument artifact.[16,17]

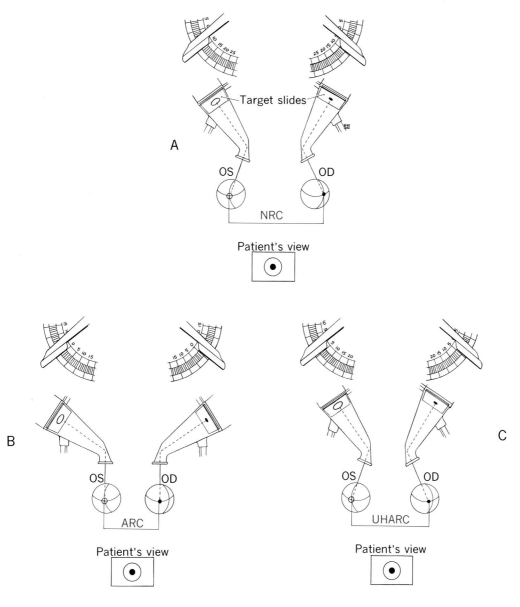

Target slides

A

OS   OD

NRC

Patient's view

B

OS OD

ARC

Patient's view

C

OS OD

UHARC

Patient's view

Figure 61

103

RETINAL CORRESPONDENCE—cont'd

Paradoxical diplopia

A patient with anomalous retinal correspondence may respond with a different type of diplopia than one would expect from the position of his eyes, since the two foveas no longer have a common visual direction. Paradoxical diplopia may occur under the following circumstances.

Figure 62

A An esotropic patient with ARC will indicate crossed diplopia when both foveas are stimulated on the amblyoscope. Similarly, an exotropic patient will experience uncrossed diplopia.

B Anomalous retinal correspondence may temporarily persist in a patient whose eyes have been straightened surgically. In this instance the fovea of the formerly deviated right eye will remain associated with a different visual direction than the fovea of the sound eye. Thus bifoveal stimulation will result in diplopia, the distance between the double images corresponding to the preoperative angle of anomaly.

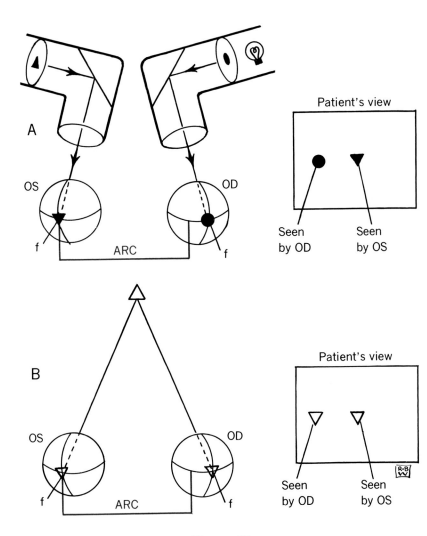

Figure 62

RETINAL CORRESPONDENCE—cont'd
Binocular triplopia and monocular diplopia

Binocular triplopia can occur under conditions of competition between normal and anomalous retinal correspondence. The essence of this phenomenon is that stimulation of a retinal area will elicit localization of the stimulating visual object in two different visual directions, corresponding to the anomalous and to the normal sensorial relationship between the two eyes. Binocular triplopia can be elicited on the amblyoscope and may occur spontaneously in the postoperative phase in patients with surgical undercorrections.

Figure 63

A Binocular triplopia in a surgically undercorrected esotrope. The visual object fixated by the fovea of OS forms an image between the fovea of the deviating eye and the retinal area that preoperatively had acquired a common visual direction with the fovea of OS. The image is localized by OD to the **right** (homonymous diplopia, in accord with NRC) and to the **left** (crossed diplopia, in accord with ARC) of the object fixated by OS.

Monocular diplopia in the nonstrabismic patient is usually caused by opacities of the media, particularly by lenticular changes. In the strabismic patient such diplopia can be elicited in an amblyopic eye with the Visuscope, or it may occur spontaneously during viewing of afterimages, or after loss of the good eye. The essence of this phenomenon is the subjective localization of one image in two different visual directions because of deep-seated anomalous retinal correspondence. Monocular diplopia may occur in foveally or eccentrically fixating amblyopic eyes.[10] Figure 63, *B*, shows monocular diplopia in a patient with eccentric fixation.

Figure 63

B The Visuscope asterisk is projected onto the fovea of eccentrically (**e**) fixating OS. The asterisk is seen by the patient as being both straight forward (corresponding to the normal principal visual direction of the fovea) and to the right (corresponding to the abnormal secondary visual direction of the fovea). The dimness of the asterisk localized normally indicates that normal foveal localization is only latently present. The latency of the normal foveal visual direction demonstrated in this manner is considered to be a good prognostic sign in pleoptics. As therapy progresses, the peripherally localized asterisk becomes dimmer and eventually disappears.

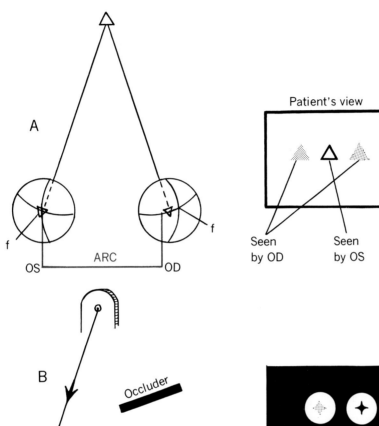

A

ARC

OS   OD

f   f

Patient's view

Seen
by OD   Seen
by OS

B

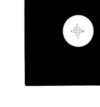

Occluder

f   e

Figure 63

107

VI. Evaluation of motor state

OVERACTING AND UNDERACTING MUSCLES

Examination of the versions in strabismic patients frequently reveals overaction or underaction of an individual muscle or of muscle groups (elevators or depressors). Overaction is usually secondary—that is, caused by weakness of the antagonist in the same eye or of the yoke muscle of the fellow eye.

More rarely, overaction is primary with a normally acting antagonist or yoke muscle. However, in some of these cases the primary paresis that has led to overaction may no longer be apparent, and secondary changes may have occurred in the overacting muscle.

Identification of overacting or underacting muscles (or muscle groups) is of paramount importance in determining the amount and type of surgery to be done.

OVERACTING AND UNDERACTING MUSCLES—cont'd

Horizontal muscles

Figure 64

A   Normal action of RLR and LMR on dextroversion.

B   Normal action of RMR and LLR on levoversion.

C   Moderate overaction of LMR.

D   Marked overaction of LMR.

E   Moderate underaction of LLR.

F   Marked underaction of LLR.

Oblique muscles

Figure 65

A   Underaction of paretic LSO.

B   Marked secondary overaction of the homolateral antagonistic LIO.

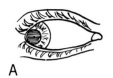

A

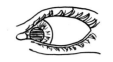

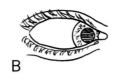

B

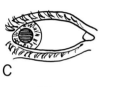

C

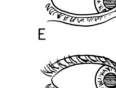

E

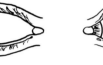

D

F

Figure 64

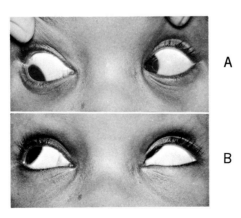

A

B

Figure 65

111

FORCED DUCTION TEST AND ITS APPLICATIONS

This test is of great value in deciding whether or not an anomaly of ocular motility is caused by mechanical factors. These may include contracture or fibrosis of a muscle, tightness of a muscle following excessive resection, shrinkage of conjunctiva or Tenon's capsule. Forced ductions should be performed before, during, and at the completion of strabismus surgery. The eye is grasped near the limbus with a forceps and *moved in the direction opposite from that in which mechanical restriction is suspected.* It is important not to press the globe into the orbit during the test, since this may simulate normal ocular motility in the presence of mechanical restrictions. When the test is done under topical anesthesia, the patient is requested to look at his hand, which is held in the direction in which the eye is being moved by the forceps. This is necessary in order to control the influence of the patient's innervation, which may otherwise counteract the passive movement of the globe and simulate mechanical restriction where none is present. In children this test is more reliable under general anesthesia, since all voluntary movements are thus excluded.

Figure 66
A Conjunctiva and episclera are grasped near the limbus with a fixation forceps.
B Eye is moved medially to test for mechanical restriction (of adduction) caused by anomalies of the lateral rectus.

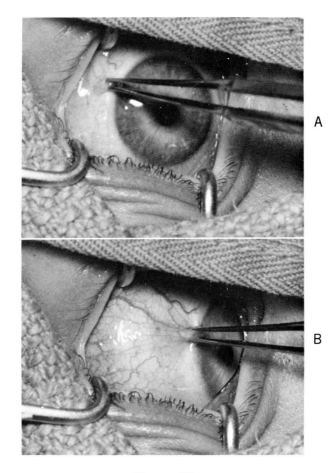

A

B

Figure 66

113

Forced duction test as an aid in differential diagnosis

Orbital floor fracture or fibrosis of the inferior rectus muscle vs. paralysis of the elevators:

Figure 67

A Resistance to passive supraduction with orbital floor fracture (shown in this drawing) or fibrosis of the inferior rectus.

B Unrestricted passive supraduction with paralysis of one or both elevator muscles.

Brown's superior oblique tendon sheath syndrome vs. paresis of inferior oblique muscle:

C Resistance to passive supraduction in adduction with Brown's syndrome.

D Unrestricted passive supraduction in adduction with paretic inferior oblique muscle.

Tight lateral rectus muscle following excessive resection operation:

E Secondary XT following surgical overcorrection of a formerly esotropic eye.

F Marked limitation of passive adduction of OS indicates tight lateral rectus syndrome. Recession or marginal myotomies of lateral rectus are indicated.

G Unrestricted passive adduction of OS. Defective active adduction indicates that recession of the medial rectus muscle was too extensive. The muscle should be advanced to its original insertion and resected.

Different causes of Duane's retraction syndrome:

H Limited passive adduction indicates fibrosis and loss of elasticity of lateral rectus muscle. If ET is present in primary position, a large recession of the medial rectus (5 to 6 mm.) is indicated that may be combined with one of the muscle transposition procedures to the lateral rectus muscle (Hummelsheim, Jensen).[18]

I Unrestricted passive adduction indicates central or peripheral neural basis of retraction, such as co-contraction of medial and lateral rectus muscles on attempted adduction (see also Figure 119). In this instance a resection of the lateral rectus muscle is contraindicated, for it may increase retraction on adduction. If there is esotropia in primary position, we recess the medial rectus 5 to 6 mm.

Thyroid myopathy of inferior rectus muscle vs. elevator paresis:

J Limited passive supraduction indicates myopathy of inferior rectus muscle.

K Unrestricted passive supraduction indicates elevator paresis.

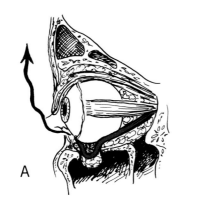
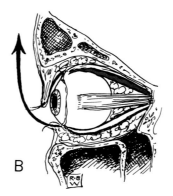

A

B

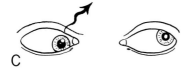
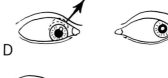

C

D

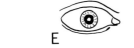
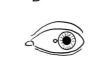

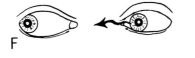

E

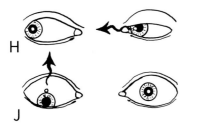
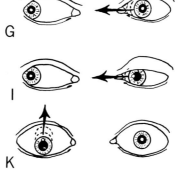

F

G

H

I

J

K

Figure 67

DIFFERENTIAL DIAGNOSIS OF ABDUCENS PALSY IN YOUNG CHILDREN

It may sometimes be difficult to establish the diagnosis of unilateral or bilateral abducens paralysis in small children. Apparent inability to abduct may be due to lack of effort involved in abducting a habitually adducted eye, unwillingness to cooperate, or weakness of the lateral rectus muscle.

Crossed fixation

Figure 68

Young children with marked esotropia (accommodative or paretic) may employ the left eye for viewing objects in the right field of vision **(A)** and the right eye to view an object in the left field of vision **(B)**. Thus no effort is made to abduct the nonfixating eye, and the patch test will differentiate between a true and a simulated abducens paralysis.

Patch test

Figure 69

A Child with a habitually deviated left eye may at first demonstrate weakness of abduction and simulate a nerve VI paralysis when the fixating eye is occluded.

B Occlusion of the fixating eye for several hours or days may demonstrate good abduction and thus differentiate between true paralysis and pseudoparalysis of the lateral rectus muscle.

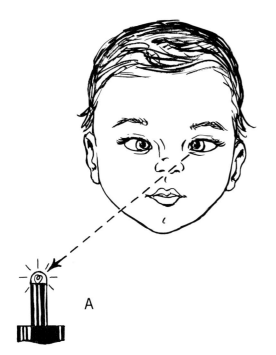
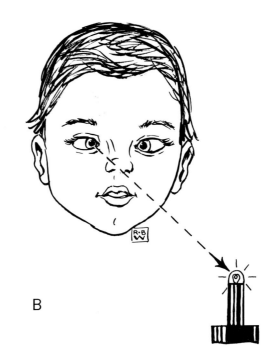

Figure 68

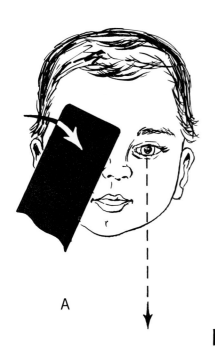
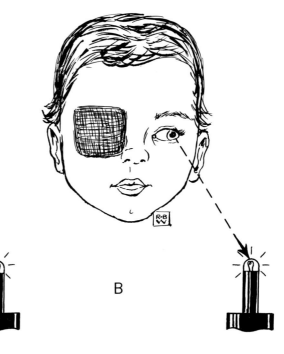

Figure 69

DIFFERENTIAL DIAGNOSIS OF ABDUCENS PALSY IN YOUNG CHILDREN—cont'd

Doll's head phenomenon

Figure 70

Sudden passive turning of the head will frequently reveal good abduction in uncooperative children and differentiate true from simulated paralysis of the lateral rectus muscle.

A Apparent weakness of abduction of either eye in an esotropic patient.

B Passive, quick turning of the patient's head reveals normal abduction OU.

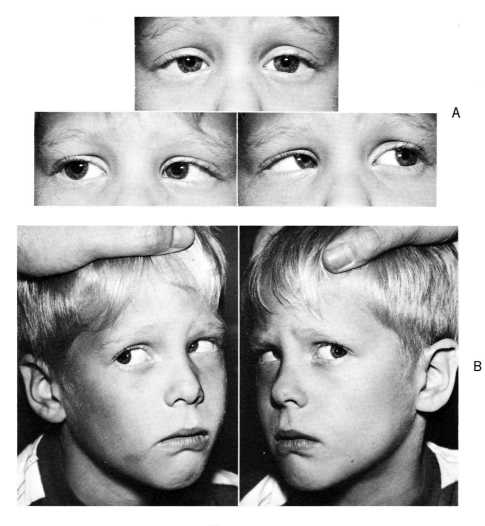

A

B

Figure 70

119

DIVERGENCE EXCESS AND SIMULATED DIVERGENCE EXCESS

When intermittent exotropia occurs during childhood, the deviation with distance fixation is often greater than at near fixation. In most instances this is due to the extremely powerful convergence tonus in children that obscures the near deviation and persists even when the eyes are momentarily dissociated by the alternate cover test. Thus it becomes necessary to differentiate between a true divergence excess and a simulated divergence excess,[19] in which the near deviation may be obscured by dynamic factors (tonic and fusional convergence). This differentiation is essential because a recession of both lateral rectus muscles is indicated in divergence excess, whereas a basic exotropia (near deviation equals distance deviation) is best treated by a resection of the medial rectus muscle combined with recession of the lateral rectus muscle of the same eye.[20] The following test indicates whether divergence excess or simulated divergence excess (basic exotropia) is present.

Patch test in simulated divergence excess:

Figure 71

A to **C** Alternate cover test reveals an exotropia that is significantly (15$^\Delta$) smaller at near than at distance fixation.

D Patch is placed over one eye for 2 to 3 hours in order to thoroughly dissociate the eyes.

E Before removal of the patch the fellow eye is covered with an occluder. After the patch has been removed, it is important to prevent the patient from using the eyes together, even momentarily, since only a brief binocular exposure may be sufficient to again obscure the near deviation by fusional convergence.

F Patch has been removed.

G and **H** If simulated divergence excess (basic exotropia) is present, rapid alternate covering will reveal a markedly increased near deviation that may match or even exceed the distance deviation, whereas with true divergence excess the near deviation will remain unchanged.

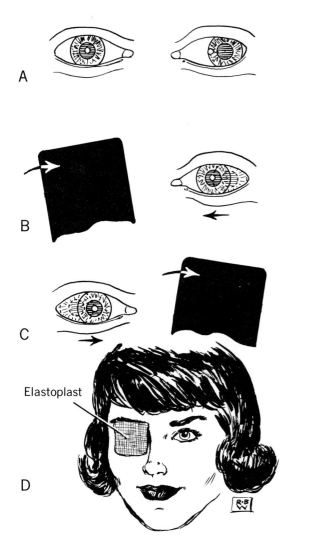

A

B

C

D

Elastoplast

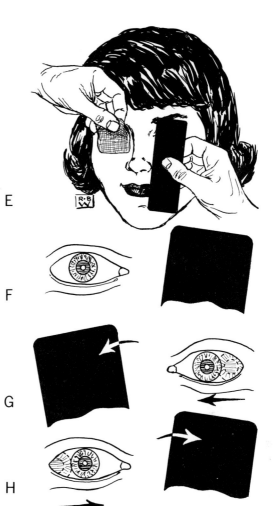

E

F

G

H

Figure 71

121

ANOMALIES OF HEAD POSITION

Anomalies of the head position may indicate a paralytic eye muscle, although they may be caused by other conditions. The head is habitually held in such a position as to avoid horizontal, vertical, or torsional diplopia. This is done so that the patient can obtain single binocular vision or, when this is not possible, peripheral fusion. In other instances the head is habitually held in the opposite position to bring about maximal separation of the double images in order to make diplopia more tolerable. Thus, the anomalous head position varies according to the nature of the sensory conditions that led to its development. Since these conditions may no longer be apparent at the time of examination, the diagnostic value of anomalous head posture for the identification of paretic muscles or muscle groups is limited. Occasionally, such an anomaly may persist, out of habit, after the ocular problem has been corrected, or because of secondary changes that have occurred in the cervical spine or the neck musculature.

Head turn (face turn)

Head turn in unilateral paralysis of a lateral rectus muscle:

Figure 72
A Head is turned into the field of action of the paralytic LLR.
B Patient utilizes the field of single binocular vision obtained on dextroversion and avoids the esotropic deviation present on levoversion.

Head turn in unilateral paralysis of a medial rectus muscle:

Figure 73
A Head is turned into the field of action of the paralytic LMR.
B Patient utilizes the field of single binocular vision obtained on levoversion and avoids the exotropia present on dextroversion.

122

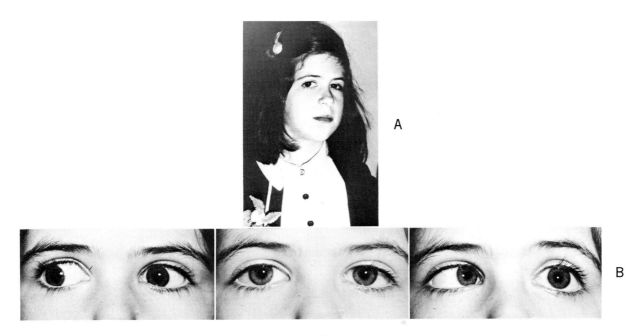

Figure 72

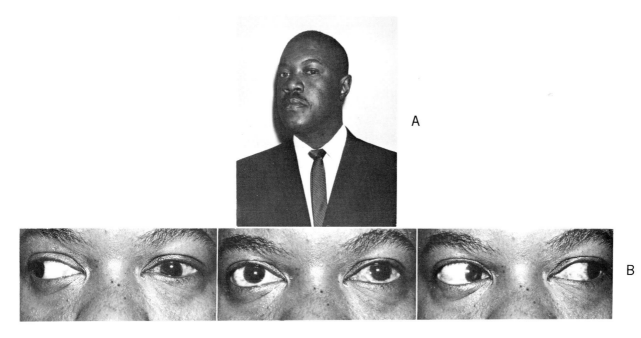

Figure 73

123

ANOMALIES OF HEAD POSITION—cont'd

Head turn (face turn)—cont'd

Head turn in paralysis of both lateral rectus muscles:

Figure 74

This patient had a congenital right paralysis of nerve VI for which she had compensated in the past by a head turn to the right. Recently she suffered a severe head injury with subsequent paralysis of the left abducens nerve. In primary position and with the head turned to either side she has constant diplopia. Occlusion of OS and head turn to the right enabled her to get around. A Jensen[18] procedure combined with a 6 mm. recession of the medial rectus muscle was performed in both eyes. The patient now has a useful field of single binocular vision, 15° abduction to each side, and diplopia only in extreme lateral gaze.

Head turn in congenital nystagmus:

The amplitude of congenital nystagmus may change in different positions of gaze. Thus visual acuity may be at its best with the eyes in a particular position.

Figure 75

A and **B** Congenital nystagmus with reduced visual acuity in primary position and on levoversion.

C The amplitude of nystagmus is reduced (or the eyes may even become steady) on dextroversion, thus resulting in an improvement of visual acuity. The patient has a head turn to the left to obtain optimal vision. A Kestenbaum procedure (resection of RMR and LLR, combined with recession of RLR and LMR) will move both eyes to the left; this will reduce the nystagmus in primary position, eliminate the head turn, and improve visual acuity.[21]

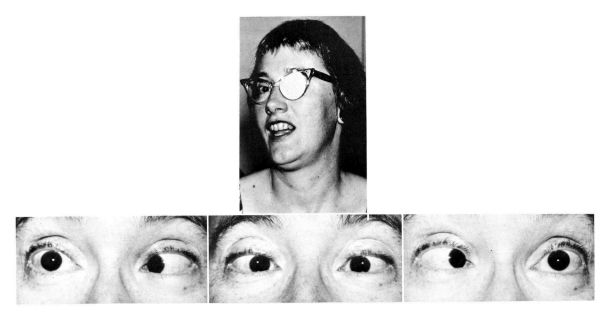

Figure 74

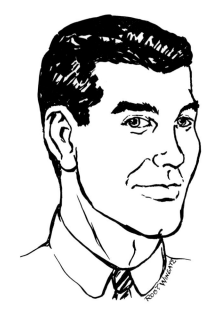

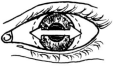

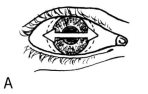

A

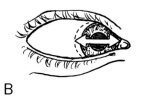

B

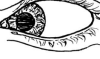

C

Figure 75

ANOMALIES OF HEAD POSITION—cont'd

Head tilt (ocular torticollis)

A head tilt (to either shoulder, around an anteroposterior axis) serves to counteract torsional diplopia in paralytic affections of the oblique and vertical rectus muscles. Head tilt is often combined with a head turn and a chin elevation or depression; it is more consistent in anomalies of the oblique than of the vertical rectus muscles. Generally, it can be said that *the head is placed in such a way as to avoid action of the affected muscle.*

Head tilt with paralysis of superior oblique muscles:

Figure 76

A Right superior oblique palsy. The face is turned and the head is tilted toward the uninvolved side; the chin is depressed. This head posture neutralizes the excycloduction of OD from the unopposed and overacting RIO, and places the eyes in a position where cooperation of the affected muscle is not required (dextroversion and elevation). For further discussion, see Figure 88.

B Left superior oblique palsy.

Head tilt with paralysis of inferior oblique muscles:

Figure 77

A Right inferior oblique palsy. The face is turned to the uninvolved side, and the head is tilted to the affected side; the chin is elevated. This head posture neutralizes the incycloduction of OD from the unopposed and overacting RSO, and places the eyes in a position where cooperation of the affected muscle is not required (dextroversion and depression).

B Left inferior oblique palsy.

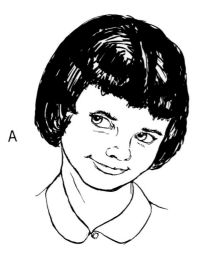
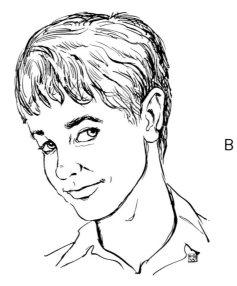

A

B

Figure 76

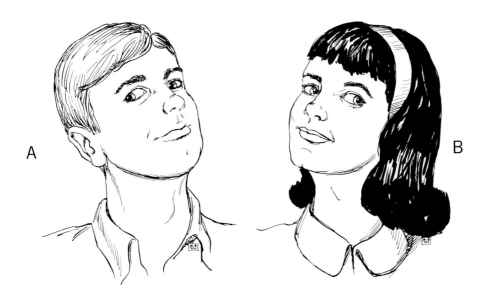

A

B

Figure 77

127

ANOMALIES OF HEAD POSITION—cont'd
Head tilt (ocular torticollis)—cont'd

Compensatory head position with paralyses of vertical rectus muscles:

Anomalies of head posture vary greatly in affections of the vertical rectus muscles, and therefore they are of very little diagnostic significance.

Head tilt with paresis of right superior rectus muscle:

Figure 78
Superior rectus paresis. The head may be turned and tilted to the involved side; the chin may be raised. In other cases the head may be tilted toward the sound side. In this instance a head tilt toward the paretic side is present and is interpreted as an effort to neutralize excycloduction produced by overaction of the yoke of the paretic muscle, the LIO.

Head tilt with paresis of left inferior rectus muscle:

Figure 79
Inferior rectus paresis. The head may be tilted to the involved or the uninvolved side, whereas the face is usually turned toward the paretic side; the chin may be depressed. In this patient no significant head tilt was present, but there was a face turn to the involved side and a slight depression of the chin to bring the eyes to a position where no cooperation of the paretic muscle was required (dextroversion and elevation).

The direction of the head tilt is fairly characteristic with paresis or paralysis of the oblique muscles: with superior oblique paralysis the head is tilted toward the uninvolved side and with inferior paralysis, toward the paretic side. With paralyses of the vertical rectus muscles the direction of the head tilt is inconsistent; the head may be tilted either toward the paretic or toward the sound side.

Analysis of the head position can be considered as only an additional diagnostic aid, and *absence of such anomalies does not exclude oblique or vertical rectus involvement.*

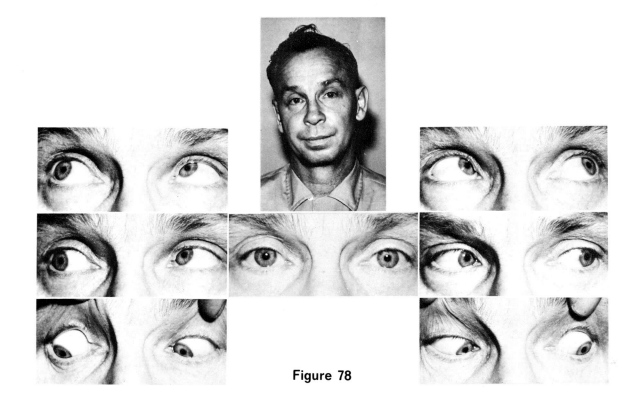

Figure 78

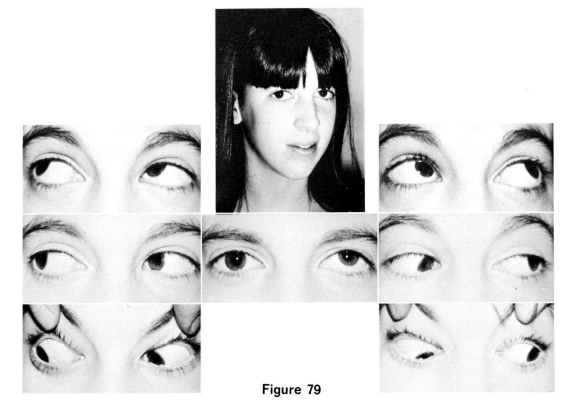

Figure 79

129

Differential diagnosis of ocular vs. congenital torticollis

Nonocular causes of torticollis in childhood include congenital bony malformations (involving those of atlas, cervical vertebrae, and ribs) or muscular malformations of the sternocleidomastoid muscle. There is marked resistance to passive straightening of the head, and a fibrous mass can often be felt in the contracted sternocleidomastoid muscle. Patching of the paretic eye relieves ocular torticollis, provided no secondary skeletal or muscular changes have developed in the neck; patching has no effect on congenital torticollis.

Congenital torticollis from fibrosis of sternocleidomastoid muscle:

Figure 80
Congenital torticollis from marked contracture and thickening of the right sternocleidomastoid muscle, which protruded beneath the skin when the head was tilted to the left shoulder.

Patch test in congenital torticollis:

Figure 81
A This patient with congenital torticollis had a comitant LHT of 5ᐞ in all positions of gaze and a marked head tilt to the left.
B A paretic vertical or oblique muscle could not be identified, and patching of either eye for several hours did not eliminate the anomalous head position. Palpation revealed a firm, thickened sternocleidomastoid muscle on the left side. The head position had been present since soon after birth.

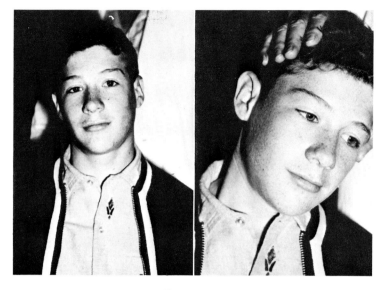

Figure 80

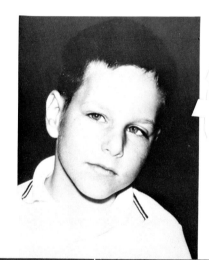

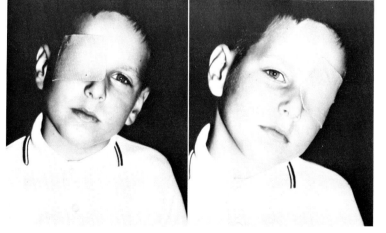

B

Figure 81

131

Differential diagnosis of ocular vs. congenital torticollis—cont'd

Patch test in ocular torticollis:

Figure 82

A Head tilt to the left in a patient with paralysis of the RSO (ocular torticollis).

B After patching of the paretic eye for 2 hours, the head tilt has disappeared.

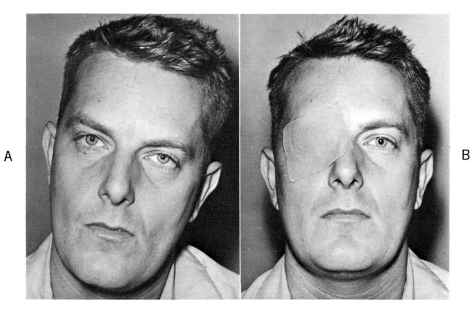

Figure 82

133

ANOMALIES OF HEAD POSITION—cont'd

Chin elevation and depression

A compensatory posture of the head resulting in elevation or depression of the chin to avoid vertical diplopia may occur as a result of paralyses of the oblique muscles or the vertical rectus muscles. Such postures may also occur with the A and V patterns in horizontal strabismus. In the latter case the purpose of the anomalous head posture is to place the eyes in a position in which the horizontal deviation is minimal or absent and fusion is possible. Chin elevation of ocular cause, but not necessarily associated with muscular anomalies, is also produced by incomplete bilateral ptosis.

Chin elevation with A esotropia and V exotropia:

Figure 83
A Chin elevation in a patient with A esotropia and fusion in downward gaze.
B Chin elevation in a patient with V exotropia and fusion in downward gaze.

Chin depression with V esotropia and A exotropia:

Figure 84
A Chin depression in a patient with V esotropia and fusion in upward gaze.
B Chin depression in a patient with A exotropia and fusion in upward gaze.

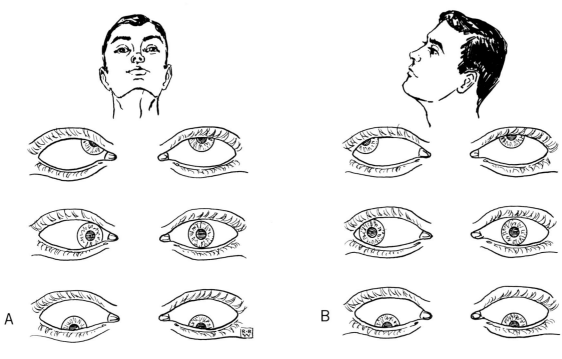

A
B

Figure 83

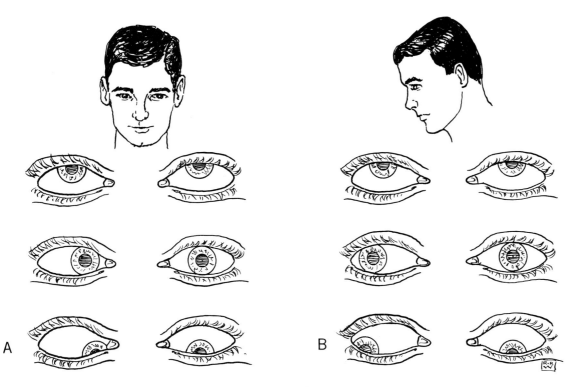

A
B

Figure 84

135

DIAGNOSIS OF VERTICAL DEVIATIONS

Ductions and versions

In cases of recent paralysis the examination of ductions and versions may be sufficient to detect the paretic muscle. Ductions are examined by covering one eye and having the fellow eye follow a fixation target in all the diagnostic positions of gaze. In this manner the field of fixation is determined and gross limitations of eye movements can be readily detected.

Although this method is often helpful in detecting complete and recent paralyses, a paresis of longer duration is easily overlooked, since with maximal innervation the eye movement may be normal in the field of the paretic muscle. Contracture of the overacting antagonist and secondary changes involving the yoke muscles of their antagonists may further obscure the primary defect; in such cases the examination of ductions is no longer useful for diagnosing the paretic muscle.

Cover comitance test

Principle: This test permits a quick qualitative diagnosis of the offending muscle in pareses of longer standing. It is based on Hering's law; that is, simultaneous and equal innervation flows to synergistic muscles. Thus if one eye is occluded, the nonoccluded eye determines the amount of innervation transmitted to the covered fellow eye. Primary and secondary deviations can be identified, and false diagnosis because of "inhibitional palsy" of the contralateral antagonist of the paralyzed muscle (Figure 15) can be avoided with this test.

Procedure: Each eye is covered alternately with an occluder held obliquely in such a manner as to permit observation of both eyes at the same time. The position of the covered eye is compared with that of the fixating eye.

Figure 85. Cover comitance test in differential diagnosis of paresis of the RSO and pseudoparesis of the LSR. The patient illustrated has a paretic RSO.

136

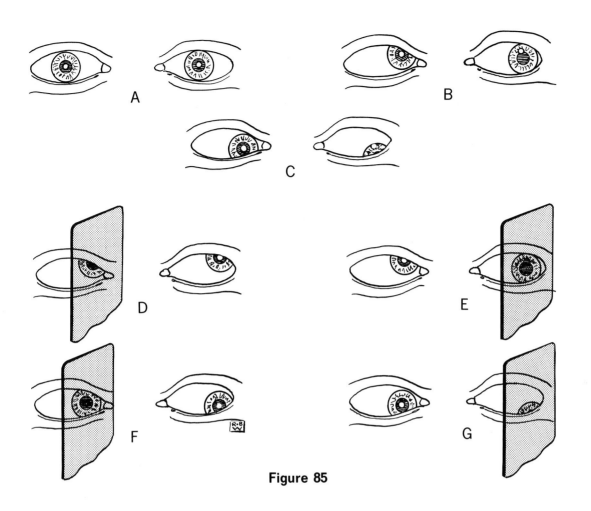

Figure 85

A When the right paretic eye is fixating, no deviation may be present in primary position.

B When looking up and to the left, an apparent paresis of the LSR may be present.

C When looking down and to the left, the right eye lags in the field of action of the RSO.

D When the right eye is covered and the left eye fixates up and left, no vertical positional difference exists between the eyes. Thus the apparent paresis of the LSR is identified as a pseudoparesis.

E Pseudoparesis of the covered left eye when the paretic eye is fixating. The antagonist of the paretic RSO, the RIO, is unopposed and thus shows marked overaction. Consequently the yoke muscle of the RIO, the LSR, will receive less than the required amount of innervation and will appear paretic.

F Lag of the paretic RSO when the nonparetic left eye is fixating (primary deviation).

G Marked overaction of the yoke muscle of the paretic muscle when the paretic eye is fixating (secondary deviation).

137

DIAGNOSIS OF VERTICAL DEVIATIONS—cont'd

Prism-cover test in diagnostic positions of gaze

For quantitative determination of the amount of vertical deviation in the field of action of each of the extraocular muscles, the prism and cover test (Figure 29) is performed in the nine diagnostic positions. The test must be performed with each eye fixating in turn. If the amount of vertical deviation changes, depending on which eye is fixating, the offending eye is easily recognized; according to Hering's law, the secondary deviation is greater than the primary deviation.

Recent paralysis of right superior oblique muscle:

Figure 86
Measurements obtained with the prism-cover test in a patient with a recent paralysis of the RSO. There is maximal deviation on looking to the left and down (the field of action of the paretic muscle) and with the paretic eye fixating.

Paresis of right superior oblique muscle of long duration:

Figure 87
Six years later the deviation has become more comitant and involves the entire field of gaze because of marked contracture of the unopposed RIO and secondary changes involving yoke muscles.

OD Fixating

—	—	RH 5△
—	—	—
—	—	**RH 30△**

R (left) — L (right)

OS Fixating

—	—	RH 5△
—	RH 5△	—
—	—	RH 15△

R (left) — L (right)

Head tilted to right: RH 35△
Head tilted to left: No vertical deviation

Figure 86

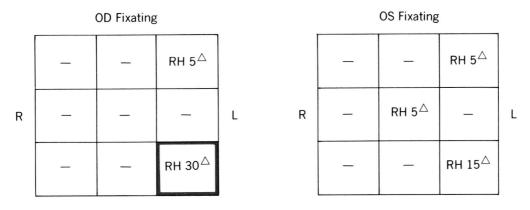

OD Fixating

RH 5△	RH 10△	**RH 25△**
RH 5△	RH 15△	**RH 20△**
RH 5△	RH 15△	**RH 30△**

R (left) — L (right)

OS Fixating

X 10△	X 5△	RH 10△
X 5△	RH 5△	RH 10△
X 3△	RH 5△	RH 10△

R (left) — L (right)

Head tilted to right: RH 35△
Head tilted to left: RH 5△

Figure 87

DIAGNOSIS OF VERTICAL DEVIATIONS—cont'd
Bielschowsky head tilt test

The previously mentioned tests may fail to detect the offending muscle in paralyses or pareses of longer standing. Because of secondary changes involving the antagonist, the yoke muscles, and their antagonists, the deviation may become increasingly comitant; then the difference between primary and secondary deviation decreases or disappears. Anomalies of the head position are not always of diagnostic help, for reasons previously mentioned. Thus the diagnosis of the offending vertical or oblique muscles must be based on their antagonistic action during supraduction and infraduction and their synergistic effect during incycloduction and excycloduction.

Physiologic principles:

Figure 88

A When the head is moved around an anteroposterior axis, compensatory eye movements occur around the anteroposterior axis of the globe because of reflex innervation originating in the otolith apparatus. Thus, when the head is tilted to the right, the right superior oblique and rectus muscles contract to provide incycloduction of the right eye. In the left eye, the left inferior oblique and rectus muscles contract to effect excycloduction of the left eye. Analogously, cycloductions in the opposite direction occur when the head is tilted to the left. The compensation of the head inclination by wheel-rotations of the eyes is incomplete and does not fully offset the angle of inclination.

B Muscles that act synergistically during cycloductions become antagonists when elevating and depressing the globes. It must be emphasized, however, that under normal conditions the vertical action of the rectus muscles exceeds that of the oblique muscles and, conversely, that the effect of the oblique muscles on cycloductions is greater than that of the vertical rectus muscles.

C When the head is tilted toward the involved side in a case of right superior oblique paralysis, the vertical and adducting action of the RSR is unopposed. Contraction of this muscle in an attempt to incycloduct the eye results in an upward movement of the right eye (positive Bielschowsky head tilt test), thus increasing the vertical deviation.

140

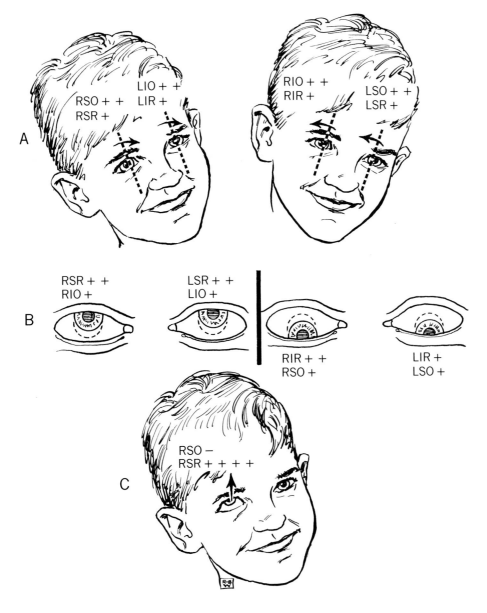

Figure 88

141

DIAGNOSIS OF VERTICAL DEVIATIONS—cont'd

Bielschowsky head tilt test—cont'd

Parks[22] pointed out that the Bielschowsky head tilt test not only identifies paretic oblique muscles but may also be employed to diagnose paretic vertical rectus muscles. He suggested the following simple three-step procedure to determine the paretic muscle:

Step I   Identify the type of hypertropia (RHT or LHT).

Step II   Identify whether vertical deviation increases on dextroversion or levoversion.

Step III   Determine whether vertical deviation increases on tilting the head toward the right or left shoulder by means of the alternate cover or cover tests.

Diagnosis of paretic muscle in patients with **right hypertropia:**

Figure 89

A   The alternate cover and uncover tests have revealed RHT. One of the following four muscles is paretic: RSO, RIR, LSR, LIO.

B   Vertical deviation increases on dextroversion, leaving two (RIR and LIO) of four possibilities (Step II).

C   **Paretic left inferior oblique.** Vertical deviation increases on tilting the head to the right because of downward movement of OS caused by the unopposed LIR, for reasons explained in Figure 88 (Step III).

D   **Paretic right inferior rectus.** Vertical deviation increases on tilting the head to the left because of upward movement of OD caused by the unopposed RIO.

E   Vertical deviation increases on levoversion, leaving two (RSO and LSR) of four possibilities.

F   **Paretic right superior oblique.** Vertical deviation increases on tilting the head to the right because of upward movement of OD caused by the unopposed RSR.

G   **Paretic left superior rectus.** Vertical deviation increases on tilting the head to the left because of downward movement of OS caused by the unopposed LSO.

142

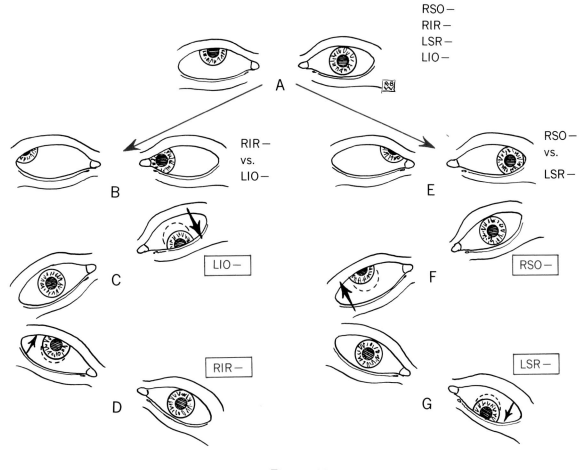

RSO –
RIR –
LSR –
LIO –

A

RIR –
vs.
LIO –

B

RSO –
vs.
LSR –

E

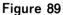 LIO –

C

RSO –

F

RIR –

LSR –

D

G

Figure 89

Figures 89 and 90 demonstrate the three-step procedure and contain all possibilities. By comparing the position of the patient's eyes with the drawings, one can identify the paretic muscle once it has been determined whether the hypertropia is on the right (Figure 89) or on the left (Figure 90). The test should be performed with the patient fixating on a distant object.

143

Diagnosis of paretic muscle in patients with **left hypertropia:**

Figure 90

A The alternate cover or the cover test has revealed LHT. One of the following muscles is paretic: RSR, RIO, LSO, LIR.

B Deviation increases on dextroversion, leaving two (RSR and LSO) of four possibilities.

C **Paretic right superior rectus.** Vertical deviation increases on tilting the head to the right because of downward movement of OD caused by the unopposed RSO.

D **Paretic left superior oblique.** Vertical deviation increases on tilting the head to the left because of upward movement of OS caused by the unopposed LSR.

E Vertical deviation increases on levoversion, leaving two (RIO and LIR) of four possibilities.

F **Paretic left inferior rectus.** Vertical deviation increases on tilting the head to the right because of upward movement of OS caused by the unopposed LIO.

G **Paretic right inferior oblique.** Vertical deviation increases on tilting the head to the left because of downward movement of OD caused by the unopposed RIR.

It must be noted that there is less vertical difference between the two eyes upon tilting the head with paresis of vertical rectus muscles than with paresis of oblique muscles. This is because the vertical action of the unopposed oblique is considerable less than that of the unopposed vertical rectus muscle.

Since Step III *always* consists of differential diagnosis between either two superior muscles (SR of one eye vs. SO of fellow eye) or two inferior muscles (IR of one eye vs. IO of fellow eye), the following simplification is helpful:

Vertical deviation increases on head tilt to same (paretic) side with paresis of Superior muscles (SO and SR).

Vertical deviation increases on head tilt to opposite (noninvolved) side with paresis of Inferior muscles (IO and IR).

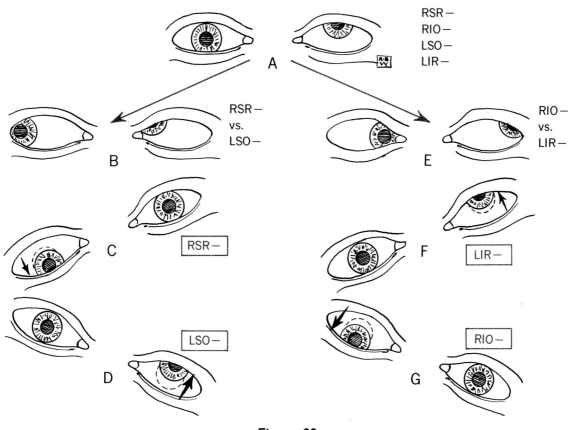

RSR—
RIO—
LSO—
LIR—

RSR—
vs.
LSO—

RIO—
vs.
LIR—

B

RSR—

C

LSO—

D

E

LIR—

F

RIO—

G

Figure 90

145

DIAGNOSIS OF VERTICAL DEVIATIONS—cont'd

Bielschowsky head tilt test—cont'd

Demonstration of head tilt test in paresis of right superior oblique muscle:

Figure 91

A Patient has an RHT (Step I; compare with Figure 89, **A**). A head tilt to the sound eye is present.

B Observation of the eyes in dextroversion and levoversion reveals an increase of the vertical deviation on levoversion (Step II; compare with Figure 89, **E**).

C Vertical deviation increases on tilting the head to the right shoulder because of unopposed action of the RSR (Step III; compare with Figure 89, **F**). If the head is tilted toward the sound left side, cooperation of the paretic RSO is not required and no vertical deviation will result.

D Examination of the versions reveals a lag of OD in the field of action of the RSO.

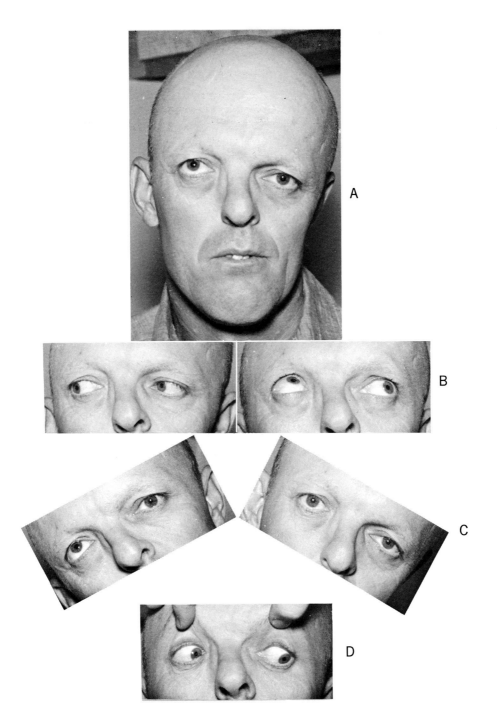

Figure 91

147

DIAGNOSIS OF VERTICAL DEVIATIONS—cont'd

Bielschowsky head tilt test—cont'd

Demonstration of head tilt test in paresis of right inferior rectus muscle:

Figure 92

A Patient has an RHT (Step I; compare with Figure 89, **A**) with pseudoptosis OS. A slight head turn and tilt to the affected side is present.

B Observation of the eyes in dextroversion and levoversion reveals an increase of the vertical deviation on dextroversion (Step II; compare with Figure 89, **B**).

C Vertical deviation increases on tilting of the head to the left shoulder because of unopposed action of the RIO (Step III; compare with Figure 89, **D**). If the head is tilted toward the right side, cooperation of the paretic RIR is not required and no vertical deviation will result.

D Examination of the versions reveals a lag of OD in the field of action of the RIR.

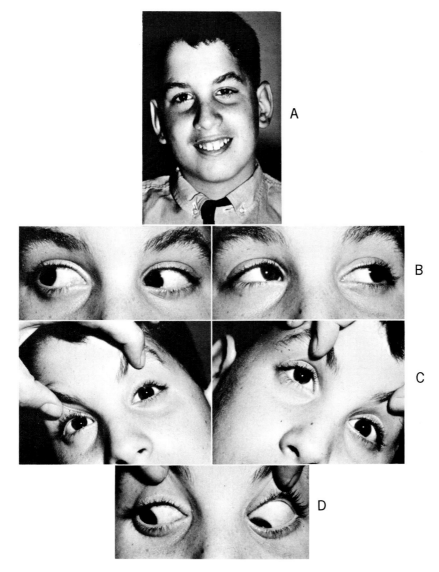

Figure 92

149

ALTERNATING SURSUMDUCTION (DOUBLE HYPERPHORIA, DISSOCIATED VERTICAL DIVERGENCE, AND OCCLUSION HYPERTROPIA)

Various terms have been employed to describe a condition that is characterized by sursumduction of each eye while the fellow eye maintains fixation. Latent nystagmus and overaction of the inferior oblique muscles are frequently, but not always, present. Occasionally, the superior obliques may be overacting.

In contrast to hyperphoria or hypertropia, in which (in the case of an RH) either the right eye is up when the left eye is fixating or the left eye is down when the right eye is fixating, either eye drifts up in this condition when the fellow eye is fixating. Consequently, a red glass before either eye will result in the red image being seen below the white one, regardless of which eye is fixating. Characteristically, the elevated eye is extorted; refixation occurs with a usually slow (tonic) infraduction that is accompanied by intorsion.

Alternating sursumduction occurs as an isolated phenomenon in patients with otherwise normal binocular function (frequently during daydreaming) or in association with other types of strabismus. It may occur in a manifest form, with both eyes open, or as latent strabismus, in which case each eye will drift up only when covered.

Figure 93

A Patient with alternating sursumduction may be orthophoric when alert and maintaining fixation on a target.

B Examinations of the versions may reveal overaction of the inferior oblique muscles.

C Occlusion of OD may result in right hyperphoria or hypertropia.

D Occlusion of OS may result in left hyperphoria or hypertropia.

E With the red glass diplopia test, the patient will see the red image below the white light regardless of whether he fixates with the right or with the left eye.

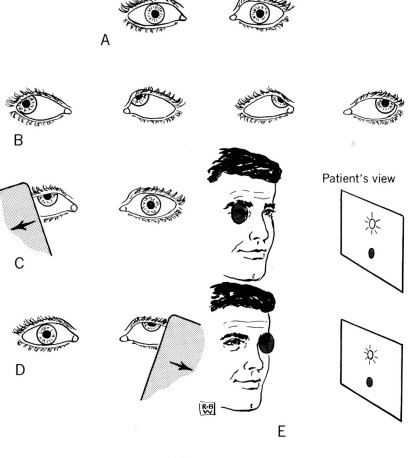

Patient's view

A

B

C

D

E

Figure 93

151

ALTERNATING SURSUMDUCTION—cont'd

Alternating sursumduction was thought by Bielschowsky to be caused by alternating and intermittent excitations of both centers for vertical divergence.[23] The fixating eye keeps its position unaltered, since the innervations of elevators and depressors neutralize each other in this eye; the nonfixating eye moves upward (dissociated vertical divergence of Bielschowsky). When the stimulation of the fixing eye is decreased, for instance by means of a neutral density filter wedge, the eye under cover may not only return from its elevated position but may actually move below the midline. Infraduction of the covered eye below the midline is very rare, however, and the existence of a supranuclear center for vertical divergence is largely hypothetical. Thus the etiology of alternating sursumduction is obscure at this time. Most authors agree that surgery is not indicated; a few have advocated a weakening procedure of the elevators.

Figure 94. Bielschowsky phenomenon in dissociated vertical divergence. A bar with neutral filters of increasing density is slowly moved before the fixating (right) eye, beginning with the least dense filter (**A**). The examiner observes the covered fellow eye, which will move downward from its elevated position, sometimes into a position of infraduction (**B**), as the stimulation of the fixating eye is decreased by filters of increasing density.

ELEVATION IN ADDUCTION (STRABISMUS SURSOADDUCTORIUS)

This condition is sometimes confused with alternating sursumduction. It is characterized by marked elevation of the adducted eye caused by primary or secondary overaction of the inferior oblique muscle(s). Right hypertropia will be present in levoversion and left hypertropia in dextroversion. Unlike findings in alternating sursumduction, the direction of the hypertropia depends on the position of gaze and hypertropia may be absent with the eyes in primary position. Association with V pattern is frequent. Surgical treatment consists of a weakening procedure (myectomy, recession) of the inferior oblique muscle(s).

Figure 95
A Marked upshoot of the adducted left eye.
B Marked upshoot of the adducted right eye.

152

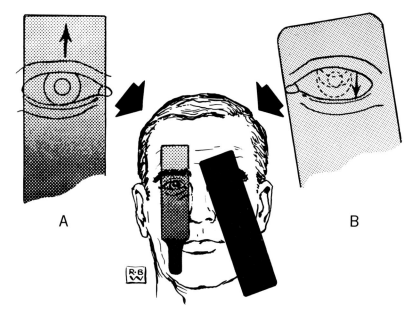

Figure 94

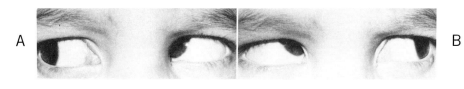

Figure 95

153

LIMITATION OF ELEVATION (DIFFERENTIAL DIAGNOSIS)

Double elevator palsy

This rare anomaly consists of combined weakness of the inferior oblique and superior rectus muscles, causing limitation of eye movements into the entire upper field of gaze.

Congenital fibrosis of the inferior rectus muscle may produce the same clinical appearance, but the forced duction test will be positive in this case.

Figure 96
Double elevator palsy with pseudoptosis OD. There is right hypotropia in primary position. Elevation OD is severely limited in primary position, abduction, and adduction. Transposition of the insertions of the medial and lateral rectus muscles to the insertion of the superior rectus muscle, as popularized by Knapp,[24] is successful when the elevation is not mechanically restricted.

Orbital floor fracture

A blowout fracture of the orbital floor following frontal contusion injury to the globe results in herniation of orbital tissue (which sometimes includes portions of the inferior oblique or inferior rectus muscle) into the maxillary antrum. Clinically, a limitation of supraduction or infraduction is present on the involved side; this may cause vertical diplopia, provided visual acuity is not severely impaired by associated injuries of the globe. Hypesthesia of the skin in an area supplied by the infraorbital nerve, enophthalmos, and positive x-ray findings are other clinical signs that may be present. The forced duction test is positive. (See Figure 67.) Surgery is indicated unless diplopia clears within 2 weeks after the injury.[25]

Figure 97
Blowout fracture of the right orbital floor. This patient had orthophoria in primary position but was unable to elevate OD above the midline in primary position, abduction, or adduction.

154

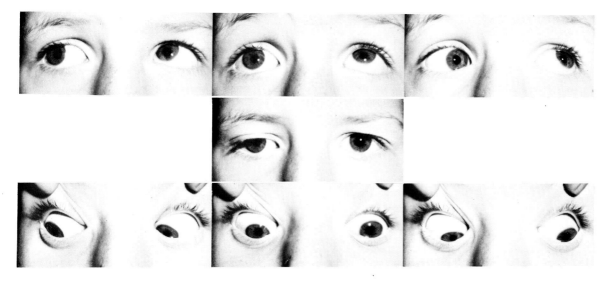

Figure 96

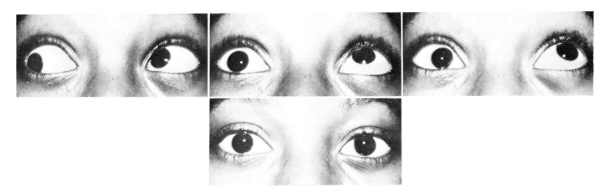

Figure 97

155

LIMITATION OF ELEVATION—cont'd

Brown's superior oblique tendon sheath syndrome

Congenital or acquired structural changes of the tendon or tendon sheath of the superior oblique muscle can limit elevation of the globe in adduction. In most instances a congenital shortening of the tendon sheath is present; however, thickening of the tendon, resulting in impaired slippage through the trochlea, or adhesions between the superior rectus and superior oblique muscles, caused by trauma or inflammation, may also produce limitation of elevation in adduction. Brown's syndrome is easily confused with paresis of the inferior oblique muscle; it is differentiated from the latter by a positive forced duction test (Figure 67).

Acquired Brown's sheath syndrome of right eye following tucking of right superior oblique muscle:

Figure 98

Marked limitation of elevation in adduction is present postoperatively. Elevation in abduction is normal. The forced duction test was positive. The etiology of this complication is not quite clear; adhesions probably play a role. This limitation of motility usually improves spontaneously with time, but it may persist in certain cases.

Acquired Brown's sheath syndrome of right eye following tenonitis:

Figure 99

A Two days after onset of pain and redness OD this patient noticed vertical diplopia on levoversion and when looking up and to the left. Ductions and versions showed limitation of elevation in adduction of the right eye. Forced ductions were positive. A subconjunctival hemorrhage developed after the forced duction test in this patient.

B Three weeks after topical therapy with corticosteroids the inflammation had subsided, diplopia had disappeared, and ocular motility was normal. Forced ductions were negative.

Congenital Brown's sheath syndrome of right eye:

Figure 100

Elevation of OD is severely restricted in adduction, limited in primary position, and normal in abduction. Surgery consisting of dissection of the sheath of the superior oblique tendon followed by temporary fixation of the eye in an overcorrected position is indicated only when a hypotropia of the involved eye is present in primary position (as shown in this case).

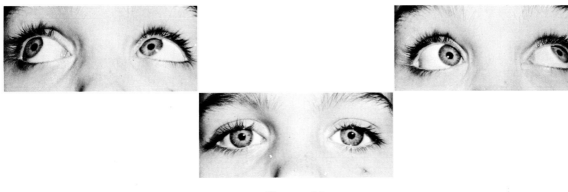

Figure 98

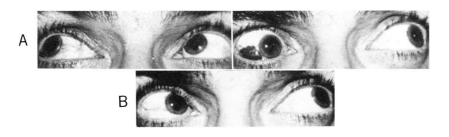

Figure 99

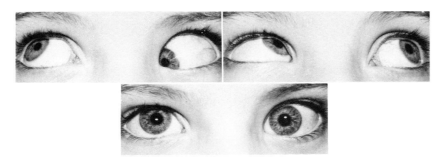

Figure 100

157

LIMITATION OF ELEVATION—cont'd
Thyroid myopathy of inferior rectus muscle

Pathologic changes may occur in the extraocular muscles with thyroid dysfunction. The histologic changes consist of lymphocytic infiltration and fibrosis of the muscle, which impair its elasticity. The inferior rectus and oblique muscles are the muscles most frequently involved. Adhesions between these muscles and adjacent orbital structures may severely impede elevation of the globe. A paralysis of the elevators is ruled out by a positive forced duction test. Maximal recession (at least 5 mm. or more) or tenotomy of the inferior rectus muscle may bring relief of vertical diplopia in primary position and downward gaze.

With endocrine myopathy of the extraocular muscles, restriction of horizontal gaze may also occur. This is either primary, and caused by edema of the medial or lateral rectus muscles, or secondary to involvement of the inferior rectus muscle.

Figure 101

A The left eye is in a constant position of infraduction and cannot be elevated to the midline in primary position, abduction, or adduction.

B After surgical exposure, a muscle hook is introduced under the LIR, but an attempt to elevate the globe by pulling on the instrument fails. This demonstrates that the defect involves the inferior rectus muscle.

C After the muscle tendon has been sectioned at its insertion, the globe can be elevated easily with a fixation forceps.

D Histologic examination of tissue obtained from the inferior rectus muscle demonstrates lymphocytic infiltration, fibrosis, and hyalinization of muscle fibers.

E Postoperative appearance after 6 mm. recession of the left inferior rectus muscle. Marked improvement of ocular motility. Note slight retraction of the left lower lid as a result of excessive retroplacement of the inferior rectus. This complication can be avoided by carefully sectioning all adhesions between the inferior rectus, Lockwood's ligament, and the lower lid.

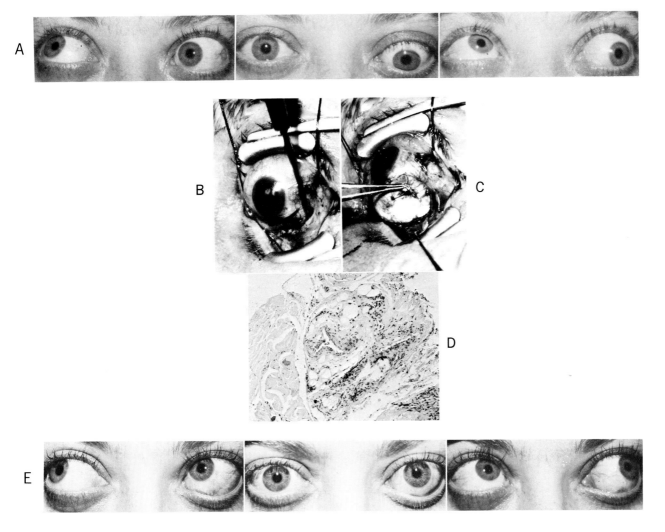

Figure 101

159

LIMITATION OF ELEVATION—cont'd
Paralysis of vertical gaze (Parinaud's syndrome)

Lesions involving the supranuclear centers (and pathways) for vertical gaze may cause paralysis of upward or downward gaze, or both. Convergence may be absent and pupillary reaction to light may be disturbed. Parinaud's syndrome is frequently seen with tumors of the pineal gland involving the superior colliculi (or their vicinity) directly or indirectly by pressure.

Figure 102

This 14-year-old girl has paralysis of voluntary vertical eye movements in addition to neurologic signs of involvement of the basal ganglia and cerebellum. A brain biopsy revealed cerebral lipidosis. The pupillary reactions are normal in this patient.

A Eyes are orthophoric in primary position. Horizontal conjugate eye movements are normal. Convergence is absent.

B An attempt to move the eyes upward innervates the frontalis muscle, but the eyes remain stationary. Similar attempts to move the eyes downward are unsuccessful.

C Full vertical excursions of the eyes on passive movements of the head (doll's head phenomenon) demonstrate that the mechanisms controlling involuntary vertical eye movements are intact.

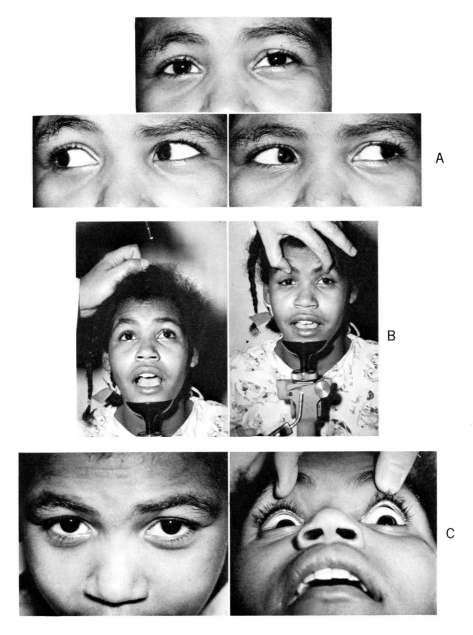

Figure 102

A AND V PATTERNS IN HORIZONTAL STRABISMUS

Measurement of the A and V patterns

Figure 103

The prism and cover test is performed at near on an accommodative target while the patient wears his full correction and with the eyes in 25° elevation, primary position, and 35° depression. If comparative measurements are to be obtained preoperatively and postoperatively, it is advisable to use a perimeter arc or a similar device with fixation targets adjustable to fixed positions of elevation and depression.[26]

V patterns

In most instances V esotropia and V exotropia are associated with overaction of the inferior oblique muscles and a primary underaction of the superior oblique muscles. In some instances the primary paresis of the superior oblique muscles is no longer detectable, and only overaction of their contracted antagonists can be demonstrated. Since the inferior oblique muscles act as abductors in upward gaze, an esotropia decreases and an exotropia increases in upward gaze when these muscles are overacting. However, anomalies of the oblique muscles cannot always be demonstrated in patients with a V pattern. Other mechanisms that have been suggested include overacting medial rectus muscles in V esotropia and overacting lateral rectus muscles in V exotropia.

Slight facial malformations are frequently *but not consistently* associated with A and V patterns: an antimongoloid slant of the lid fissures may be associated with overacting inferior obliques in V esotropia and with underacting inferior obliques in A exotropia. Conversely, a mongoloid lid fissure is often found with overacting inferior obliques in V exotropia and underacting inferior obliques in A esotropia.[27]

Mechanism:

Figure 104

A Marked overaction of inferior oblique muscles results in excessive abduction in upward gaze. Decreased abduction in downward gaze is due to underacting superior oblique muscles.

B Versions reveal overacting inferior oblique muscles.

162

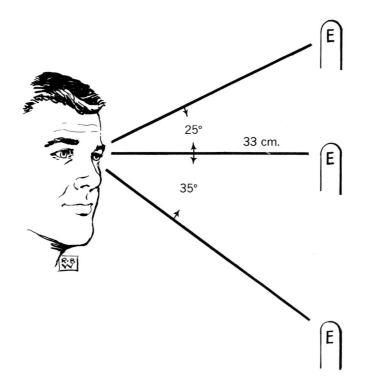

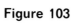

25°

33 cm.

35°

Figure 103

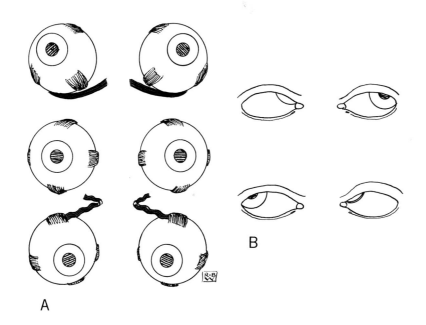

A

B

Figure 104

163

A AND V PATTERNS IN HORIZONTAL STRABISMUS—cont'd

V patterns—cont'd

V esotropia:

Figure 105

Downward (antimongoloid) slant of the lid fissures. The deviation measured 35$^\Delta$ ET in downward gaze and 5$^\Delta$ ET in upward gaze. Versions demonstrate overaction of the RIO and underaction of the RSO.

V esotropia with chin depression:

Figure 106

This patient has normal lid fissures in the presence of a marked V esotropia. The deviation measured 40$^\Delta$ ET in downward gaze and 10$^\Delta$ ET in primary position. Orthophoria was present in upward gaze, and the patient held his chin depressed when doing close work. Versions reveal overaction of both inferior oblique muscles and underaction of the RSO.

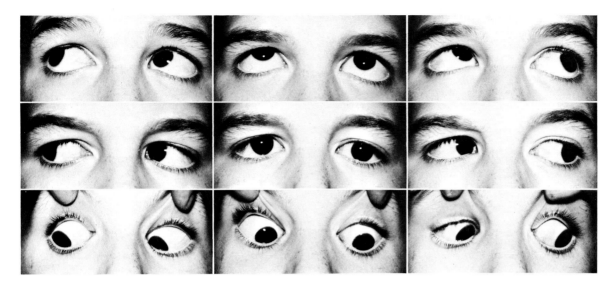

Figure 105

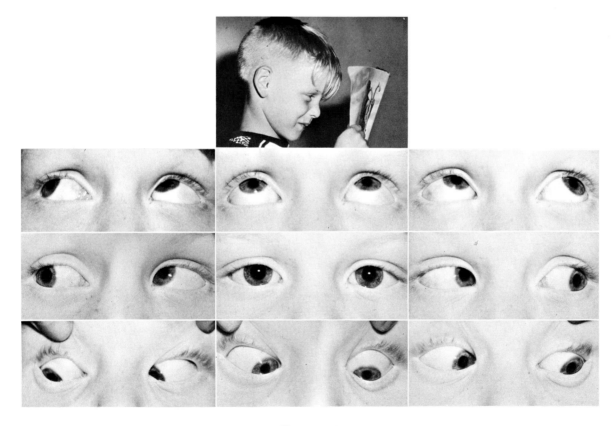

Figure 106

165

V patterns—cont'd

V exotropia:

Figure 107

Downward (antimongoloid) slant of lid fissures. The deviation measured 15ᐃ XT in downward gaze, 20ᐃ XT in primary position, and 40ᐃ XT in upward gaze. Versions reveal overaction of both inferior oblique muscles and slight underaction of both superior oblique muscles.

Management:

V esotropia: When there is overaction of the inferior oblique muscles, myectomy of these muscles in combination with (or to be followed by) horizontal surgery is indicated. When there is normal action of the inferior oblique muscles, either horizontal surgery alone or recession of one or both medial rectus muscles with downward transposition of their insertions is indicated. (See Figure 112.) This may be combined with resection of the lateral rectus and supraplacement of its insertion. When there is orthophoria in primary position and a small ET in downward gaze, temporal transposition of the inferior rectus muscles or infraplacement of the medial rectus muscles (without recession) is recommended.

V exotropia: When there is overaction of the inferior oblique muscles, myectomy of these muscles in combination with (or to be followed by) horizontal surgery is indicated. When there is normal action of the inferior oblique muscles, horizontal surgery alone is indicated. When the deviation is small in primary position or downward gaze, a recession of both lateral rectus muscles should be combined with upward transposition of their insertions (Figure 112).

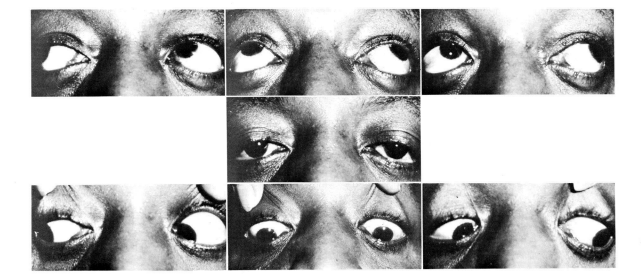

Figure 107

A AND V PATTERNS IN HORIZONTAL STRABISMUS—cont'd
A patterns

In most instances overaction of the superior oblique muscles can be demonstrated. This may or may not be combined with underaction of the inferior oblique muscles. Since the superior oblique muscles act as abductors in downward gaze, esotropia decreases and an exotropia increases in downward gaze when these muscles are overacting.

However, anomalies of the oblique muscles cannot always be demonstrated in patients with an A pattern. Underacting lateral rectus muscles have been said to cause A esotropia, and underacting medial rectus muscles to produce A exotropia.

Mechanism:

Figure 108

A Marked overaction of the superior oblique muscles causes excessive abduction in downward gaze; the inferior oblique muscles are underacting. For a better view of the action of the superior oblique muscles as abductors see Figure 4.

B Versions reveal overaction of superior oblique muscles.

A esotropia:

Figure 109

Upward (mongoloid) slant of lid fissures. The deviation measured 30△ ET in downward gaze and primary position and increased to 45△ ET in upward gaze. Versions demonstrate marked overaction of the RSO and less overaction of the LSO. There is underaction of the RIO.

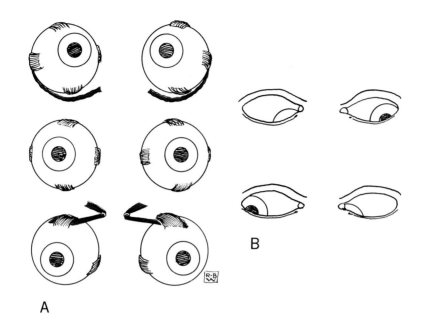

A

B

Figure 108

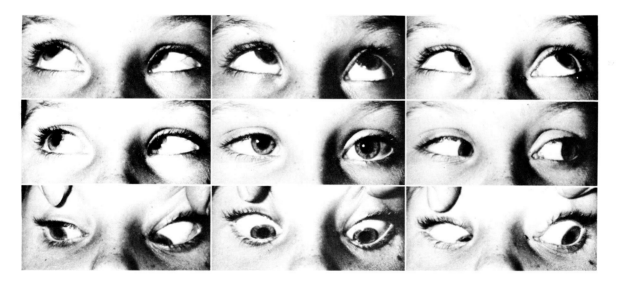

Figure 109

169

A patterns—cont'd

A exotropia:

Figure 110

Orthophoria in upward gaze; the deviation increased to 40$^\triangle$ XT in primary gaze, and to 45$^\triangle$ XT in the downward position of gaze. It is of interest that overaction of the superior oblique muscles could not be demonstrated in this patient.

Management:

A esotropia: No surgery is indicated when there is only a small angle of esotropia in primary position and below. With marked overaction of the superior oblique muscles and an angle in primary position (and below) of sufficient size to warrant surgery, a bilateral tenectomy of the superior oblique muscles is recommended in combination with (or to be followed by) horizontal surgery. With normal action of the oblique muscles, horizontal surgery is indicated; it may be combined with upward displacement of the medial rectus and/or downward displacement of the lateral rectus muscle. (See Figure 113.)

A exotropia: When there is overaction of the superior oblique muscles, they should be tenectomized in combination with (or to be followed by) horizontal surgery. When the oblique muscles are normal, horizontal surgery is indicated, either alone or combined with downward transposition of the lateral rectus muscle (Figure 113) and/or upward transposition of the medial rectus muscle.

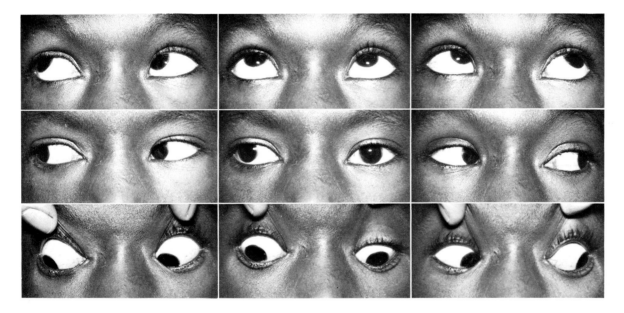

Figure 110

Transposition of horizontal rectus muscles in treating the A and V patterns

As stated before, when an A or V pattern occurs without anomalies of the oblique muscles, the effect of horizontal surgery can be enhanced in one direction of gaze or diminished in another direction by transposing the muscle insertion vertically (usually not more than one muscle width) in combination with or without the conventional strengthening and weakening procedures.

This surgical method is based on the fact that the horizontal effect of the medial and lateral rectus muscles changes in favor of a vertical and wheel-rotational effect when the eye is elevated or depressed from the primary position. For instance, when the eye is elevated, the medial rectus will become less of an adductor and more of an elevator and excycloductor. This is because the muscle plane (determined by the center of rotation of the globe and the centers of origin and insertion of the muscle) will change. Similarly, with the eye depressed the action of the medial rectus will change from adduction to depression and incycloduction.

The muscle is transposed in that vertical direction in which its horizontal function should be further weakened and in the direction opposite from that in which one wishes its horizontal function to be more effective.

Vertical transposition of horizontal rectus muscles may be performed in conjunction with symmetric surgery (recession or resection of both medial or lateral rectus muscles, respectively) or with a combined recession-resection on one eye.

Figure 111
A With the globe in elevation the medial rectus muscle becomes less of an adductor and more of an elevator.
B In depression the medial rectus muscle acts more as a depressor and less as an adductor.

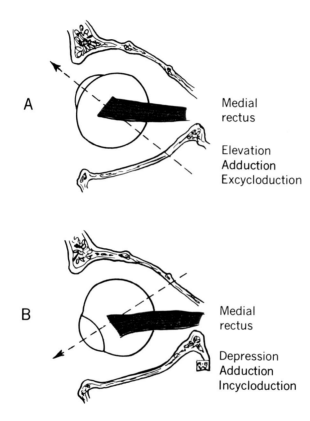

A   Medial rectus

Elevation
Adduction
Excycloduction

B   Medial rectus

Depression
Adduction
Incycloduction

Figure 111

Transposition of horizontal rectus muscles in treating the A and V patterns—cont'd

Figure 112

A Infraplacement of the medial rectus further weakens its adductive power in depression (where the deviation is largest in a V esotropia).

B Supraplacement of the lateral rectus increases its abductive function in depression by changing its muscle plane.

Figure 113

A **The V pattern.** It is easy to remember that the medial rectus should be transposed "toward the apex of the pattern" and the lateral rectus "away from the apex of the pattern." In V esotropia the medial rectus is infraplaced (and recessed); the lateral rectus is supraplaced (and resected). In V exotropia, lateral rectus recession is made more effective by moving the insertion upward; a medial rectus resection is made more effective by moving the insertion downward.

B **The A pattern.** In an A esotropia, perform upward displacement of the medial rectus muscle(s) ("toward the apex of the pattern") with recession; with an A exotropia, use downward displacement of the lateral rectus muscle(s) with recession.

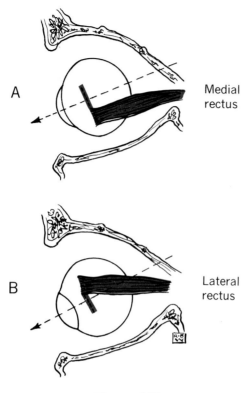

A

Medial
rectus

B

Lateral
rectus

Figure 112

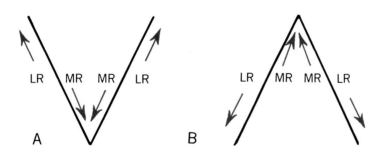

A

LR   MR   MR   LR

B

LR   MR   MR   LR

Figure 113

175

VII. Some forms of strabismus

ACCOMMODATION AND ESOTROPIA

Accommodation in uncorrected hyperopia

An uncorrected hypermetropic refractive error elicits an increased accommodative effort in order to maintain a clear image on the retina at near and distance fixation.

Figure 114
A In hypermetropia the rays emitted by a distant object converge toward a point located behind the retina (3 D hypermetropia).
B The image of the distant object can be focused on the retina by an accommodative effort (3 D accommodation at distance fixation).
C At near fixation (33 cm.) the eye not only has to accommodate the 3 D required for this distance but also has to compensate for the refractive error by additional accommodation (3 + 3 = 6 D of accommodation at near fixation).

Accommodation is closely linked with the convergence mechanism; increased central demands for accommodation will call for an increase of convergence innervation (accommodative convergence). Thus uncorrected hypermetropia may lead to esophoria or esotropia unless the increase of accommodative convergence is offset by the fusion mechanism (relative fusional divergence). Such esodeviation is eliminated by prescription of the hyperopic correction if the strabismus is purely refractional in nature.

176

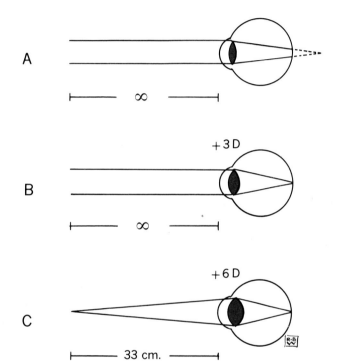

A

∞

B

+3 D

∞

C

+6 D

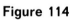

33 cm.

Figure 114

177

ACCOMMODATION AND ESOTROPIA—cont'd

Effect of glasses on accommodative esotropia

Figure 115

A Excessive accommodation in an uncorrected hypermetropia of 3 D and excessive accommodative convergence uncompensated for by relative fusional divergence have led to an esodeviation at near fixation.

B Photograph of a patient with accommodative esotropia.

C Correction of the hyperopic refractive error leads to straightening of the eyes.

D Effect of +3 D spherical glasses in a patient with corrected hypermetropia.

Effect of miotics on accommodative esotropia

The effect of glasses can be simulated by circumventing the central linkage between accommodation and accommodative convergence. This is accomplished by the action of anticholinesterase drops that potentiate neuromuscular transmission at the ciliary body synapses.[28] An effort to accommodate will elicit less synkinetically associated convergence. Accommodative esotropia can thus be favorably influenced.by phospholine iodide and similar drugs that facilitate accommodation and thereby reduce accommodative convergence.

Miotics are indicated to eliminate small-angle esotropia after surgery in patients undergoing orthoptic therapy, to rule out an accommodative component in an esotropic infant prior to surgery, in patients with a high AC/A ratio, and in surgically overcorrected intermittent exotropia.

Figure 116

A Esotropia before miotics.

B Orthophoria with miotics.

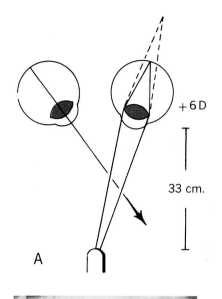

+6 D

33 cm.

A

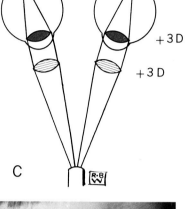

+3 D

+3 D

C

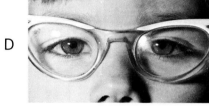

B

D

Figure 115

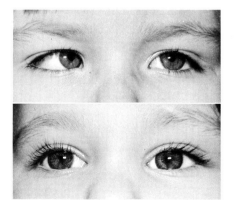

Figure 116

179

AC/A ratio

Whether or not an increased accommodative effort causes an esotropia depends not only on the degree of uncorrected hypermetropia and the effectiveness of compensatory fusional mechanisms but also on the ratio between accommodative convergence and accommodation (the AC/A ratio). Normally, the amount of convergence associated with accommodation has a mean value of 4; that is, $4^\triangle$ of accommodative convergence is associated with 1 D of accommodation. For a given amount of accommodation some patients have a greater or lesser degree of associated accommodative convergence (high or low AC/A ratio). For instance, a patient with a *low* AC/A ratio and 3 D uncorrected hypermetropia may not develop an esodeviation, since there is less than normal associated accommodative convergence at near fixation; but a *high* AC/A ratio may cause esotropia in patients with only minimal uncorrected hyperopic refractive errors (or even in emmetropes) since there is more than normal accommodative convergence associated with accommodation. For the same reason, residual esotropia may be present at near fixation after correction of the distance deviation by means of glasses. In such instances additional plus lenses in a bifocal lower segment (or miotics in addition to the glasses) may be helpful. The AC/A ratio does not depend on refractive errors, heterophoria, and heterotropias. It cannot be altered by orthoptics, and there is debate as to whether this relationship may remain fixed throughout life.

The determination of the AC/A ratio is a valuable clinical procedure. Rather than calculation of the AC/A by comparing the near and distance measurements of strabismus we prefer the more accurate lens gradient method. With the refractive error fully corrected the near deviation is measured with the prism and cover test while the patient reads 20/20 letters at 33 cm. distance. Measurements are repeated with plus and minus 3.00 spherical lenses over the patient's glasses. The accommodative convergence is thus determined over a range of 6 D accommodation.

For a more refined measurement it is necessary to exclude the influence of fusional convergence by measuring the AC/A on the amblyoscope with special slides and lenses inserted to cover the full range of accommodation.[29]

Effect of bifocals in esotropia with high AC/A ratio

Figure 117

A Orthophoria through glasses at distance fixation. For technical reasons the eyes were slightly elevated while this and the following photographs were taken.

B An esotropia remains at near fixation.

C Plus 3 D spherical bifocal segments decrease the accommodative effort at near fixation and thus lessen the associated accommodative convergence. The eyes are orthophoric when looking through the lower segment.

Bifocals should be prescribed only when the patient has an esodeviation of less than $5^\triangle$, or has orthophoria at distance fixation and changes from esotropia to esophoria at near fixation when looking through additional plus lenses. The strength of the bifocals must be titrated by selecting the minimal plus correction that allows the patient to fuse. *In children it is important that the upper edges of the bifocal segments bisect the pupils.*

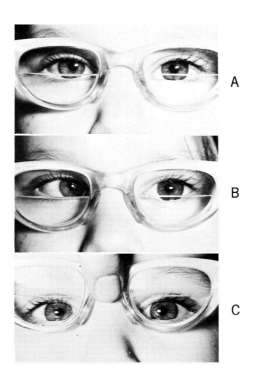

Figure 117

CONVERGENCE SPASM

Occasionally, a convergence spasm may simulate an esotropia at near fixation. Sustained convergence is usually associated with a spasm of accommodation; it can occur with hysteria. The pupils are miotic and the induced myopia causes decreased visual acuity at distance.

Figure 118. Convergence spasm simulating esotropia.
This 34-year-old female patient with a hysteric personality complained of episodes of diplopia at near fixation.

A At distance fixation an intermittent exotropia of $20^\triangle$ was present.

B At near fixation on an accommodative target, the eyes suddenly went into a position of overconvergence. This was associated with complaints of diplopia and with bizarre nodding movements of the head.

C The convergence spasm persisted for 8 to 10 minutes after removal of the near fixation target.

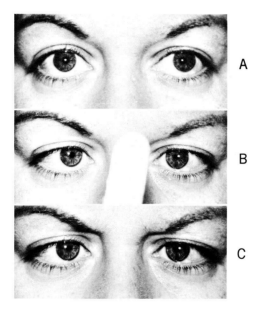

A

B

C

Figure 118

183

DUANE'S RETRACTION SYNDROME

Duane's retraction syndrome is characterized by limitation of abduction, retraction of the globe on attempted adduction, and narrowing of the palpebral fissure on adduction. Frequently, the adducted eye moves into a position of elevation; less frequently, the eye moves downward. This syndrome occurs more often in the left eye; it can be bilateral and hereditary. Possible etiologic factors include fibrosis of the lateral rectus muscle, with a resultant inelastic fibrous band, or paradoxical innervation because of anomalous peripheral or internuclear connections. In the latter cases it has been shown that there is co-contraction of the medial and lateral rectus muscles on attempted adduction, resulting in retraction of the globe. On attempted abduction the lateral rectus muscle is not innervated; this has been documented electromyographically. For diagnosis and treatment see Figure 67.

Figure 119. Duane's syndrome.
A No anomaly is present in primary position.
B Abduction OS is limited.
C Palpebral fissure narrows; the globe retracts and moves into a position of extreme elevation on attempted adduction.
D Lateral view of palpebral fissure with the eye in primary position.
E Narrowing of the palpebral fissure and marked retraction of the globe on attempted adduction.

STRABISMUS FIXUS

Figure 120
Occasionally, extremely large deviations occur in patients with bilateral abducens paralysis and maximal contracture of the medial rectus muscles. The medial rectus muscles may be (or become) totally replaced by fibrous tissue. It is impossible to abduct either eye across the midline, even with forced ductions.

Treatment consists of maximal (at least 6 mm.) recession of both medial rectus muscles combined with recession of conjunctiva and Tenon's capsule to the semilunar fold, 10 mm. resection of both lateral rectus muscles, and temporary fixation of the globes with sutures in a position of abduction.

184

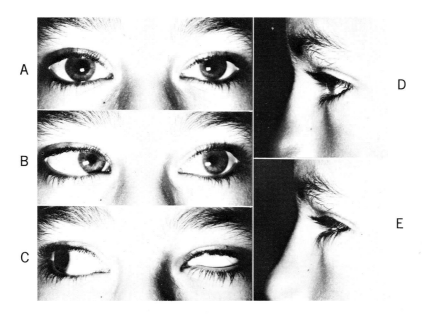

Figure 119

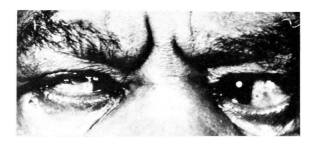

Figure 120

185

NERVE III PALSY

Figure 121. Incomplete paralysis of nerve III of left eye.
This patient developed paralysis of nerve III following a skull fracture 3 years before. The pupil of the left eye is fixed; partial ptosis is present in the primary position. Examination of the versions revealed complete paralysis of the LIO and LSR and paresis of the LMR and levator palpebrae muscles. Because of paralysis of both elevators, a left hypotropia is present in primary position and in upward gaze.

ABERRANT REGENERATION OF NERVE III

Figure 122

A In primary position a partial ptosis of the left upper lid is present because of paresis of the levator muscle.

B On downward gaze the left upper lid rises. This is thought to be due to regeneration of nerve fibers, originally connected with the inferior rectus, that have grown into the sheath of the nerve fibers supplying the levator muscle. Because of the resemblance of this phenomenon to lid retraction on downward gaze in thyroid dysfunction (Graefe's sign), it has been called "pseudo Graefe's sign."

C Adduction of the affected eye in upward gaze caused by aberrant regeneration of superior rectus fibers that have become connected with the medial rectus. Pupillary constriction may occur in adduction but was not present in this case.

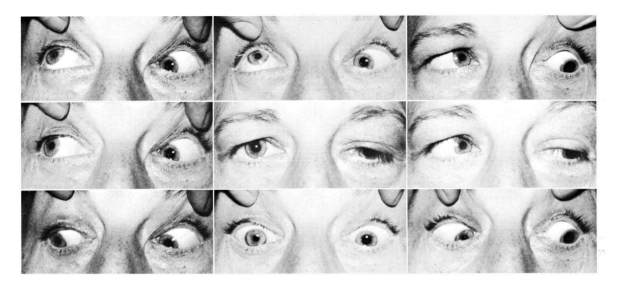

Figure 121

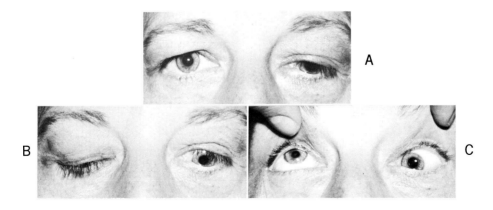

A

B

C

Figure 122

187

OCULAR MYOPATHY (CHRONIC PROGRESSIVE OPHTHALMOPLEGIA EXTERNA)

This condition is characterized by slow and progressive paralysis of all the extraocular muscles. In the final stage both eyes are virtually immobile in the orbits, although they can be passively moved on forced ductions. Ptosis may or may not be associated. The pupils are spared. Opinions are divided as to the cause of this disease, which is thought to be due to nuclear degeneration or to a primary disease of the muscle itself. Ocular myasthenia is differentiated from this condition by the Tensilon test.

Figure 123
Ocular myopathy in a 63-year-old man. Inability to move the eyes into any direction of gaze.

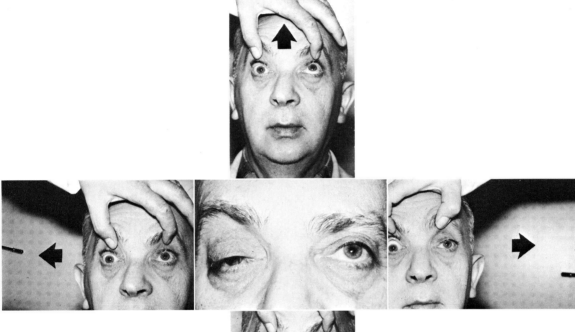
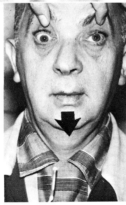

Figure 123

MARCUS GUNN (JAW-WINKING) PHENOMENON

This rare congenital anomaly is characterized by ptosis and momentary lid retraction upon opening the mouth or moving the jaw to the opposite side. An anomalous connection is present between the nuclei of the external pterygoid and of the levator muscle. The surgical therapy has recently been reviewed by Iliff.[30]

Figure 124. Marcus Gunn phenomenon in a 12-year-old girl.
A Ptosis of the left upper lid.
B Lid retraction upon opening the mouth.
C The lid opens farther when the jaw is moved to the uninvolved side.
D No effect by movement of jaw to the involved side.

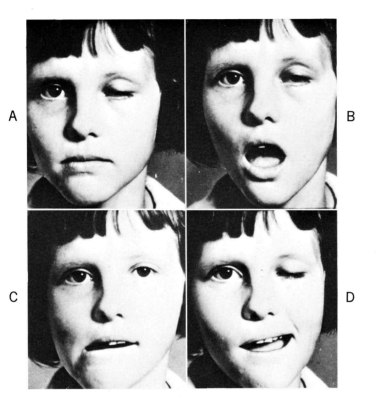

Figure 124

References

1. Boeder, P.: Co-operative action of extra-ocular muscles, Br. J. Ophthalmol. **46:**397-403, 1962.
2. Jampel, R. S.: The fundamental principle of the action of the oblique ocular muscles, Am. J. Ophthalmol. **69:**623-638, 1970.
3. von Noorden, G. K., and Mackensen, G.: Phenomenology of eccentric fixation, Am. J. Ophthalmol. **53:**642-661, 1962.
4. Romano, P. E., and von Noorden, G. K.: Limitations of the cover test, Am. J. Ophthalmol. **72:**10-12, 1971.
5. Romano, P. E., and von Noorden, G. K.: Atypical response to the four-diopter prism test, Am. J. Ophthalmol. **67:**935-941, 1969.
6. Swan, K. C.: The blind spot mechanism in strabismus. In Allen, J. H., editor: Strabismus ophthalmic symposium II, St. Louis, 1958, The C. V. Mosby Co.
7. von Noorden, G. K., and Maumenee, A. E.: Clinical observations on stimulus deprivation amblyopia (amblyopia ex anopsia), Am. J. Ophthalmol. **65:**220-224, 1968.
8. von Noorden, G. K., and Burian, H. M.: Visual acuity in normal and amblyopic patients under reduced illumination. I. Behavior of visual acuity with and without neutral density filter, Arch. Ophthalmol. **61:**533-535, 1959.
9. von Noorden, G. K., Allen, L., and Burian, H. M.: A photographic method for the determination of the behavior of fixation, Am. J. Ophthalmol. **48:**511-514, 1959.
10. von Noorden, G. K.: The etiology and pathogenesis of fixation anomalies in strabismus, Am. J. Ophthalmol. **69:**210-245, 1970.
11. Lang, J.: Evaluation in small angle strabismus or microtropia. In International Strabismus Symposium at Giessen in 1966, Basel, 1968, S. Karger.
12. Parks, M. M.: The monofixational syndrome, Trans. Am. Ophthalmol. Soc. **67:**601-657, 1969.

13. Helveston, E. M., and von Noorden, G. K.: Microstrabismus: a newly defined entity, Arch. Ophthalmol. **78**:272-281, 1967.
14. Bagolini, B., and Capobianco, N. M.: Subjective space in comitant squint, Am. J. Ophthalmol. **59**:430-442, 1965.
15. Cüppers, C.: Grenzen und Möglichkeiten der pleoptischen Therapie. In Hollwich, F., editor: Schielen-Pleoptik-Orthoptok-Operation, Stuttgart, 1961, Ferdinand Enke.
16. Romano, P. E., von Noorden, G. K., and Awaya, S.: A re-evaluation of diagnostic methods of retinal correspondence, Am. Orthopl. J. **20**:13-21, 1970.
17. Awaya, S., von Noorden, G. K., and Romano, P.: Anomalous retinal correspondence in different positions of gaze, Am. Orthopl. J. **20**:28-35, 1970.
18. Jensen, C. D.: Rectus muscle union: a new operation for paralysis of the rectus muscles, Trans. Pac. Coast Otolaryng. Ophthalmol. Soc. **45**:359-387, 1964.
19. Burian, H. M.: Exodeviations: their classification, diagnosis and treatment, Am. J. Ophthalmol. **62**:1161-1166, 1966.
20. von Noorden, G. K.: Divergence excess and simulated divergence excess: diagnosis and surgical management, Doc. Ophthalmol. **26**:719-728, 1969.
21. Cooper, E. L., and Sandall, G.: Surgical treatment of congenital nystagmus, Arch. Ophthalmol. **81**:473-480, 1969.
22. Parks, M. M.: Isolated cyclovertical muscle palsy, Arch. Ophthalmol. **60**:1027-1035, 1958.
23. Bielschowsky, A.: Lectures on motor anomalies, Hanover, N. H., 1956, Dartmouth Publications.
24. Knapp, P.: The surgical treatment of double elevator paralysis, Trans. Am. Ophthalmol. Soc. **67**:304-323, 1969.
25. Emory, J. M., von Noorden, G. K., and Schlernitzauer, D. A.: Orbital floor fractures: long-term follow-up of cases with and without surgical repair, Trans. Am. Acad. Ophthalmol. Otolaryng. **75**:802-812, 1971.
26. von Noorden, G. K., and Olson, C. L.: Diagnosis and surgical management of vertically incomitant horizontal strabismus, Am. J. Ophthalmol. **60**:434-442, 1965.
27. Urrets-Zavalia, A., Jr., Solares-Zamora, J., and Olmos, H. R.: Anthropological studies on the nature of cyclovertical squint, Brit. J. Ophthalmol.
28. Breinin, G. M.: Accommodative strabismus and the AC/A ratio, Am. J. Ophthalmol. **71**:303-311, 1971.
29. Sloan, L. L., Sears, M. L., and Jablonski, M.: Convergence-accommodation relationships, Arch. Ophthalmol. **63**:283-306, 1960.
30. Iliff, C. E.: The optimum time for surgery in the Marcus Gunn phenomenon, Trans. Am. Acad. Ophthalmol. Otolaryng. **74**:1005-1009, 1970.

Index

198